D1538799

# INTRODUCTION TO
# CLINICAL SUPERVISION

## IN

# SPEECH PATHOLOGY

# INTRODUCTION TO
# CLINICAL SUPERVISION
## IN
# SPEECH PATHOLOGY

GEORGE W. SCHUBERT, Ph.D.

*Professor of Speech Pathology*
*Chairman, Department of Speech and Audiology*
*Dean, University College*
*University of North Dakota*
*Grand Forks, North Dakota*
*Bush Summer Fellow, 1976*
*Bush Foundation, St. Paul, Minnesota*

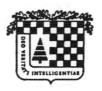

WARREN H. GREEN, INC.
St. Louis, Missouri, U.S.A.

GALLAUDET COLLEGE LIBRARY
WASHINGTON, D. C.

616.8
538i
1978
c.1

**Dedicated to:**

Arline Florance
Kathleen Jane
Cheryl Lynn

219279

*Published by*

WARREN H. GREEN, INC.
8356 Olive Boulevard
St. Louis, Missouri 63132

*All rights reserved*

© 1978 by WARREN H. GREEN, INC.

*Library of Congress No. 77-81799*

*ISBN No. 87527-162-6*

*Printed in the United States of America*

## PREFACE

This book is written in an effort to provide historical information to the reader in the area of Clinical Supervision and to provide guidance and procedures for completing the difficult task of clinical supervision. It is nearly impossible for any single text to provide all of the possible procedures which have been and are presently being employed by clinical supervisors. Many factors dictate the supervisor's behavior. Some of these factors are the age of the client, the intelligence of the client, and the type of speech disorder. Obviously, there are some other factors which also serve to limit the supervisor's repertoire. This book does not address itself to each individual factor, but procedures which can be used in their present form or which can be adopted to be used in supervision.

Many of the ideas have been passed on to me by my professional colleagues. All of these people in that way share in this book.

This book reflects the position of the author regarding clinical supervision. This position is that quality supervision leads to improved clinical skills and that these skills are as important as academic knowledge and training in research procedures.

GEORGE W. SCHUBERT

# INTRODUCTION

This book reflects the many different approaches and concepts involved in the complex process called Supervision of Practicum Experience in Speech Pathology. Clinical supervision has often been referred to as the "step-child" to our profession. However, the material included within this book is an effort to remove the stigma that clinical supervision is a "step-child" or a "reluctant profession."

Procedure and rationale for methods used by clinical supervisors are presented. The book is prepared for clinical supervisors, students involved in practicum experiences and other professional clinicians who wish to evaluate and improve their clinical skills.

The book is divided into nine chapters, each one discussing a different segment of the clinical supervision process. It is interesting to note that material included within some of the chapters has been used for many years as part of the clinical training process. Chapter 1, The Supervisor, defines and describes the clinical supervisor. Qualification, responsibilities and guidelines for the supervisor are presented. Decision making procedures and the importance of knowledge of the decision making process are related to the clinical supervisory process.

Chapter 2, The Lesson Plan, presents and discusses the importance of lesson plans for student clinicians and professionals. Procedures for writing, developing and evaluating lesson plans are presented.

Chapters 3 and 4 deal with the evaluation and grading of student clinicians. Historical information is included regarding observation systems. The Analysis of Behavior of Clinicians (ABC) System is presented in detail. Collection data and analysis forms for the use of the system are included. Discussion is presented concerning letter grading and the pass-fail system of grading in clinical practicum courses. Criteria for evaluating and modifying student clinician behavior is discussed.

Report Writing, Chapter 5, examines the importance of communicating relevant information when writing reports. The do's and don't's of report writing are included.

Most clinical supervisors use some type of conference when advising student clinicians. Chapter 6, titled The Supervisor-Supervisee Conference, examines the function of the conference. Specific behaviors which can be identified during the supervisory conference are identified and discussed. Information regarding the length of the conference is presented. Also, a brief description of *The Underwood Category System for Analyzing Supervisor-Clinician Behavior* is included in this chapter.

Use of Videotape and Closed Circuit Television in Clinical Supervision, Chapter 7, points out the advantages of using videotapes and closed circuit television for supervision. Uses of these procedures for other than clinical supervision are also reviewed. The development and use of a videotape library is discussed.

Nonverbal communication, its use and value as part of therapy and supervision, is revealed in Chapter 8. Even though research regarding the use of nonverbal behaviors is in its infancy in speech pathology and audiology, the topic must be addressed. How and when nonverbal cues are used and recent studies in this area are reviewed. The definitions and use of the terms most often used with nonverbal behaviors, are discussed.

Supervision of Supportive Personnel, Chapter 9, the last chapter in the book, examines such things as: The purpose of communication aides; guidelines which have been established when communication aides are employed; and the supervision of aides. Problems which can be anticipated and success which has been achieved with communication aides are topics discussed in this chapter. Each chapter is concluded by five question or issue statements for discussion purposes.

# CONTENTS

# INTRODUCTION TO
# CLINICAL SUPERVISION
## IN
# SPEECH PATHOLOGY

# *CHAPTER 1*

## THE SUPERVISOR

### Defined

The clinical supervisor is a professional who is responsible for the growth, improvement and development of clinical skills of student-clinicians. The supervisor is an evaluator of clinical competencies and in the final stages of the student's training becomes a colleague of the student-clinician.

### Qualifications of the Supervisor

The clinical supervisor is an important element of the speech clinician's training program. In a broad sense, the supervisor must have an understanding of human relationships and the ability to empathize with people. The effective supervisor is a recognized leader and is respected by his colleagues and students. The supervisor must have a positive and dynamic approach toward learning. Also, he should be democratic in his approach toward working with people.

The qualities of a clinical supervisor in speech pathology can be identified. Five general qualities which the clinical supervisor must possess are:

— A sincere interest in the profession

— A sincere interest in helping students gain professional skills

— A sincere interest for the care and treatment of clients

— A sincere interest for self-improvement

— Professional competence

3

Any person who is interested in becoming a clinical supervisor in speech pathology and cannot meet all of these five general criteria should not become a member of a group which places such demands on its professionals. Clinical supervisors need to be dedicated to their profession and need to receive internal rewards for their commitment and dedication to working with student-clinicians and clients.

The clinical supervisor must be able to perform the following tasks:

— Be able to serve as a resource person for the student-clinician.

— Be able to help the student-clinician establish appropriate goals and objectives for the client.

— Be able to evaluate goals and objectives established for the client.

— Be able to interpret and evaluate diagnostic information.

— Be able to help the student-clinician analyze his own behavior, thereby teaching the student-clinician to become a self-evaluator.

— Be able to analyze the behavior of the student-clinician.

— Be able to be objective and unbiased in his evaluations.

— Be able to recognize and accept the many individual differences among people.

— Be able to help the student gain self-confidence in his clinical skills.

— Be able to establish goals for each student-clinician.

— Be able to serve as an advisor in record keeping and report writing.

— Be able to be consistent when making recommendations and be sure to discuss the "whys" of the recommendations made.

— Be able to recognize the weak areas of the student clinician's background and to provide experiences which will modify this situation.

— Be able to encourage creativity.

— Be able to help the student integrate theory into practice.

— Be able to reduce the amount of direct advice as the student clinician gains experience and confidence.

— Be able to encourage the student clinician to utilize a variety of materials and procedures.

— Be able, during the final stages of therapy, to establish a feeling of colleagueship between the clinician and supervisor.

— Be able to record systematically data regarding the clinician's behavior and to establish appropriate goals.

— Be able to create and maintain an atmosphere where learning can take place.

— Be able to observe therapy often enough to be fully acquainted with all aspects of the clinician and client.

— Be able to present himself as a model for clincians to view. However, he should not present himself as the perfect or only model.

— Be able to be flexible and tolerable.

Obviously, the aforementioned items are not an exhausted listing of qualities of a clinical supervisor. It is essential, however, that a supervisor have each and every one of these behaviors.

## Historical Information

A review of the professional literature which pertains to qualifications of a clinical supervisor is very limited and would be close to nonexistent if it were not for professionals who have become interested in this area during the last ten years.

Halfond (1964) points out that one outstanding lack in training in speech pathology is in the supervisory aspect of clinical practicum. It is pointed out that the aspect of clinical supervision is either downgraded or neglected. The author also notes that neither special competence nor training of the clinical supervisor is required.

Miner (1967) in one of the most comprehensive reports concerning the clinical supervisor set forth eight guidelines for quality supervision. The guidelines are as follows:

1. Understanding and utilizing the dynamics of human relationships which promotes the growth of the student clinician.

2. Establishing realistic goals with the student clinician which are clearly understood by both student and supervisor.

3. Observing and analyzing the teaching-learning act involved in the therapy procedures.

4. Providing the student with the necessary "feedback" which will enable him to become increasingly self-analytical.

5. Knowing and using a variety of materials, methods, and techniques which are based on sound theory, successful practice, or documented research.

6. Recognizing and setting aside the supervisor's personal prejudices and biases which influence perception and develop rigidity in order that the subjective task of evaluation may become as objective as possible.

7. Challenging and motivating the student clinician to strengthen his clinical competency without the supervisor's assistance.

8. Appreciating the individual differences among student clinicians to such an extent that supervisory programs and practices may be radically altered to suit his needs.

Schubert (1974) suggested that minimal requirements be established for a person to serve as a clinical supervisor. Schubert felt that just because the supervisor was certified by the American Speech and Hearing Association this did not qualify him to supervise all kinds of cases. Therefore, he suggested the following eight minimal requirements for supervisors:

— A Master's degree in the subject area in which supervision will be administered

— Certificate of Clinical Competence in the Subject area in which supervision will be administered

— Two hundred hours (internship) of practicum in supervision under the direction of a certified and experienced supervisor; The practicum should be with a wide variety of clinicians.

— Practicum experiences as a supervisor, involving supervision of a wide range of clients with different disorders

— Two years of paid professional experience following the completion of the Clinical Fellowship Year

— Knowledge of and experience with a wide variety of diagnostic tests and instruments within the subject area or areas in which supervision is to be administered

— Basic knowledge in scientific methodology; be able to plan, supervise, evaluate systematically controlled clinical research

— Six credit hours of academic course work specifically designed to prepare students to work actively as a clinical supervisor

It is important to note that these are suggested minimal requirements. Another qualification which the clinical supervisor should have is specialized training in the area of clinical supervision. This may be in the form of short courses, workshops and academic and practicum course work. Also, knowledge in the area of counseling is extremely useful. This is important because the clinical supervisor must communicate, and communicate effectively with a wide variety of people who have different backgrounds and personalities. The clinical supervisor must be able to be diplomatic, yet direct and firm; also, he must be able to yield and to show empathy. Although a clinical supervisor possesses knowledge, it is worthless unless he is able to convey this knowledge to the people he must communicate with.

### Present Status of the Supervisor

Although it is easy to paint a bleak picture of the clinical supervisor by reviewing and examining changes during the past few years, there is also a bright side.

The clinical supervisor is one of the hardest working persons in the training setting. Often he is supervising by 8:00 a.m. and leaving the clinic sometime after 5:00 p.m. Most of the nine-hour day at the clinic is devoted to direct supervision and conferencing with students. The evening hours of the clinical supervisor are occupied with evaluating reports, evaluating lesson plans, and completing other paper work.

Although the clinical supervisor may lack some important clinical and indepth training, there is no one more dedicated to the profession than the clinical supervisor. Although dedicated, the clinical supervisor is often the poorest equipped person on the departmental faculty to handle the important job of clinical supervision.

In a comprehensive study conducted by Schubert and Aitchison (1975), much was learned about the clinical supervisor. They found that the typical clinical supervisor in a university or college training program is represented as follows: This person is a female between the ages of twenty-six and thirty-two years of age. She has been employed in her present position from one to three years and is employed in a nine to ten month a year job. Her present salary is between $9,000 and $12,000 for the nine to ten months. She holds a Master's degree in speech pathology and is certified by the American Speech and Hearing Association.

This typical supervisor worked as a clinician for three to five years before becoming a supervisor and had no academic course work to help prepare her as a clinical supervisor.

In her professional setting, the clinical supervisor works in an institution which is accredited by the American Speech and Hearing Association, but she does not receive tenure.

In her direct role as a supervisor, she supervises students at all levels of their clinical practicum experience. She does not have a caseload of her own, but does do demonstration therapy. The supervisor is assigned to supervise eleven to fifteen different clients per week. The supervisor is assigned ten to fifteen student clinicians to supervise weekly.

The supervisor uses videotapes, audiotapes, post-therapy conferences, lesson plans and objective evaluation systems in completing the supervisory task. Of these, post-therapy conferences and lesson plans are used most often with audiotapes being used least often.

## The Supervisor as a Decision Maker

A decision maker is one who processes information with the intent to answer a question or select a particular outcome. So, in effect, all people are decision makers. Some decisions are very easy to make, others are complex and require much thought and a great deal of time. The more complex the problem, the greater the necessity to use some type of plan as a formal decision making process.

The clinical supervisor is a decision maker of the highest level. He is making decisions continually about both the clinician and the client. To do this effectively, the supervisor needs an orderly system of processing information.

The supervisor, in making his decision, should be careful to use the following steps:

- identify the problem
- obtain necessary information

   note possible solutions
- evaluate possible solutions
- develop a plan for implementing solution selected
- develop a procedure for the evaluation of the solution selected

It is useful to follow the above steps when making a clinical decision. It gives the supervisor a feeling of confidence. This confidence comes from the knowledge that a formal plan has been followed, and the supervisor understands how the decision has been reached. Confidence also comes from the important fact that the supervisor knows his plan includes evaluation of the solution he selected.

There are many personal factors which can influence the supervisor when making decisions. Some of these include how much clinical experience the supervisor has had, how many different kinds of cases the supervisor has supervised, and how many student clinicians the supervisor has supervised. Additional factors which contribute to the supervisor's decision making skills regarding practicum are the different environments in which the supervisor has been employed and the background the supervisor has from his associations with his fellow supervisors and other colleagues.

Two additional factors which influence a supervisor when making decisions are his use of ingenuity and his imaginative or creative ability. The supervisor who has more ingenuity and is more creative will intuitively incorporate these factors when problem solving. This supervisor will make different kinds of recommendations to students than will the supervisor who is less creative and less imaginative. This does not mean that one supervisor is right and one is wrong; it means that two different people are problem solving and making recommendations according to their own assets and liabilities.

With most decisions the supervisor must take into account a changing environment. People change in their ages, their interests, their friends, their living environments, and many other things. These factors which change must be taken into account as the decision is made.

An important factor in making decisions is one of time. A supervisor will find that with some decisions only minutes are available for making a decision. In this case, the analysis is usually less formal. However, if the supervisor is in the habit of using formal decision making criteria when making complex decisions, he can apply much of this information to the immediate situation. Limited time is a factor which can reduce the number of alternatives one has to choose from. A limited amount of time or lack of the necessary amount of time can force a supervisor into a poor or incorrect decision. When this situation exists, the decision to make no decision should be used, if it is a possible choice. Of course, this in itself is a decision.

An appropriate amount of time is necessary to collect information and to verify that the information is correct and accurate. We know that mistakes are made on reports. We know that what people say and what the listener thinks they say are often quite different. Information must be checked for accuracy. This is needed to evaluate the alternatives to a decision and to evaluate the consequences of each alternative. Additional time is then needed to select and implement the decision.

The amount of time it takes to implement a particular decision needs to be of concern to the supervisor. For example, a supervisor may decide that a clinician (Clinician A) does not have enough experience and knowledge to work with Client A and wants to assign Clinician B to Client A. However, Clinician B, because of his present competence, will have a full caseload for two more weeks. From the above example we can examine the factors which the supervisor needs to take into account.

— Experience of Clinician A

— Experience of Clinician B

— Client's needs

— Possible consequences of Clinician A continuing to work with the client for two additional weeks

— Effect the termination of working with the client may have on Clinician A or on the client

— Other possible alternatives

In this case, the supervisor may delay implementing the change for two weeks. As long as Clinician A is making some progress with the client and is not harming the client in any way, the supervisor may decide to delay the change in clinicians until Clinician B can treat the client.

A supervisor learns how to make correct decisions through the use of practice with formal procedures and by having expertise and confidence in his professional area. The possession of these three factors by a supervisor will create a decision maker who is likely to make the correct decision. The supervisor, as a decision maker, should keep the following statement in mind: a problem clearly stated is already half solved. All too often an inexperienced decision maker attempts to solve a problem or makes a decision without identifying and isolating the problem.

## Summary

The skills and background of clinical supervisors vary to a great extent. However, there appear to be common elements which a clinical supervisor should possess. These criteria are: a sincere interest in the profession, the student, and the client; be professionally competent; and a desire for self-improvement. The clinical supervisor must serve as a resource person, be able to establish appropriate goals and objectives for the clinician and client, and be able to correctly evaluate these goals and objectives. The supervisor must be able to be objective and unbiased and help the student gain self-confidence and become a self-evaluator. He must be consistent in his behavior, encourage creativity and encourage the use of a variety of procedures to complete the task of supervision.

The typical supervisor is a young female who works between nine and ten months a year for a modest salary. She is certified by the American Speech and Hearing Association. This supervisor supervises cases with a variety of speech disorders and is responsible for approximately twelve student clinicians.

Although the clinical supervisor may be ill-prepared according to today's standards, he is a dedicated, overworked professional person who is growing in status annually.

The clinical supervisor is a decision maker and should be knowledgeable about the decision making process. The decision maker needs to take into account such things as time, environment, accuracy of information, correct identification of the problem, liabilities and assets of the decision maker, plan for implementing a decision, implementation of the solution, and procedures for evaluating the decision when making a decision. Decision making experience and knowledge of using a formal plan are beneficial to the growth and development of the supervisor.

## Questions and Issues

1. All people who are certified by ASHA as Speech Pathologists should not function as clinical supervisors. If you believe this statement to be true, support your position; if you believe the statement to be false, support that position.

2. Qualifications of a clinical supervisor are numerous. What do you think are the five most important qualifications a supervisor can possess? Why?

3. In what way and to what degree do you think the role of the clinical supervisor will change in the next five years?

4. What value is the knowledge of a formal decision making process to the clinical supervisor?

5. What is meant by the statement "the supervisor has integrity?"

# CHAPTER 2

## LESSON PLANS

### Introduction

Lesson plans can be defined as maps or directions for future growth. Lesson plans guide and direct the clinician regardless of the degree of experience or preparation. It is nearly impossible to progress in the desired direction without lesson plans. Initial thought must be given to planning objectives, goals, and procedures for the therapy session. This chapter will include answers to several questions regarding the what, how, why, where, when and who of lesson plans.

### What Is a Lesson Plan?

A lesson plan is a guide in varying amounts of detail. The lesson plan maps out the future work for the clinician and the supervisor. A lesson plan serves as a directory for the supervisor. It might be called a menu, if this analogy is desired. First, the supervisor can determine what entrés are offered. The objectives are there to give substance to the lesson. An objective must be developed before a clinician can conduct therapy satisfactorily. It must be determined in what direction he will go. To try to do therapy without an objective in mind usually leaves one quite disappointed. The supervisor should always insist upon several objectives. Remember, it is the responsibility of the supervisor to attend to progressive therapy without tangents. Only clearly thought out objectives can lead in that direction.

Second, objectives without activities well thought out and planned in advance by the clinician are like salads without a main dish, rather unfilling in their rewards. Many activities are fun but ineffective in their end results. The activities planned by the

14

clinician and supervised by the supervisor should be fun, easily understood, and an aid to the clinician in reaching his goal. Often activities are out of sequence because in discussions the clinician heard it mentioned, heard it was successful, and tried it; only to find that the activity was too advanced or too difficult for his client. Several activities should be included because what might work one time will not work at another. Let it be added here that a separate lesson plan should be written for each client, remembering each individual is 'unique, and the problem each has is also unique. Lesson plans should be modified and improvised for each client. One source of frustration for both clinician and supervisor is, "It worked before, why not now?" Don't allow this pitfall; cover it before it opens into a chasm of bad habits for the beginning or student clinician.

When activities are planned in advance, materials can be selected and set aside. There is nothing more discouraging or disgusting than to go to the supply area, try to select materials and supplies, and find that the necessary things are gone, broken, or in some instances, dismantled. Thought and preparation before the session can sooth and relax a clinician and client. If the few minutes before a session with a client are rapid and frustrating, the clinician enters the therapy session nervous and up tight. The client perceives this, and the session is off to a bad beginning. It is good for all concerned if the first few minutes are relaxed.

Preparing materials in advance also prepares the clinician. The physical preparation of the therapy room is important, but equally as important is the mental preparation of the clinician. Many clients are seen in the course of therapy time, and the clinician must spend some time considering each client separately. Therefore, as the clinician chooses and selects materials for activities, he is thinking about that particular client. Often the clinician finds that one client is more difficult to prepare for and in determining this he allows more preparation time. A clinician and supervisor are naive if they think that a clinician does not have to prepare mentally and emotionally for each clinical session. The excitements and frustrations experienced by the clinician often must be placed aside and forgotten for the time. Personal feelings often interfere with therapy if the clinician has not prepared himself mentally.

Once the materials and supplies are gathered together, it is necessary that they be placed (ahead of time) in the therapy room in an inconspicuous manner so as not to distract from the other duties of the clinician prior to the performance of the activity. If the materials and supplies are not placed in the room ahead of time, or if they are not organized in the order of their use, much valuable learning time is lost. Plus, the break in therapy may cause the client to have a break in attention. It then may follow that the client will not cooperate with the clinician and the activity will fail. Not because the activity was poor or inadequate, but because the clinician was unprepared or unorganized. Mental and physical organization are necessities when dealing with the speech handi-capped person.

We have now had the entre', salad, proper preparation of our meal, and it is now dessert time. As in all menus, the desserts are the end to all good things. The comparison then continues by con-sidering the evaluation as the dessert. The evaluations by both clinician and supervisor serve as the conclusion to a lesson. This may not be present. If this be the case, again one may be left wanting. A brief evaluation leaves one satisfied and content. The evaluation serves to conclude the session, and it provides the opportunity for both clinician and supervisor to remark on the experiences before they are forgotten. It is difficult to remember in any detail the success or failure of any activity a day or even hours later, particularly if subsequent therapy with another client has intervened. Observations must be recorded, if any lesson plan is to be successful. Some activities or actions should be repeated because they were successful; others should be modified or eliminated because they were inappropriate and did not reach the expected level of satisfaction. The evaluation of the day's activities does not need to be lengthy or elaborate. It should be sufficiently detailed to be useful. Observations should be objective, but also feelings should be included. If the feelings of the clinician are not noted, they will soon be forgotten and it is impossible to objectively record feelings after the session has been over for any length of time.

A lesson plan is then a guide or menu for the day's activities. Without a lesson plan the day's activities would be unorganized and undeveloped. The therapist would be working in an irregular, impromptu manner rather than in a spontaneous, smooth fashion for the benefit of all.

### Who Needs a Lesson Plan?

A lesson plan is a necessary tool of therapy. It is important to all involved in building a satisfactory and productive therapy session. The clinician, the supervisor, and the client all are affected either by its presence or by its absence.

The clinician needs the lesson plan for guidance and advancement. Even though the clinician writes the plan, he needs to use it to guide him through his therapy session. It would be extremely difficult for a clinician to remember what activities were planned, what materials were necessary, and what exact objectives were to be met on a particular day with a particular client if it were not for lesson plans. The clinician has many other things on his mind, and he sees many clients in a day. These all tend to necessitate lesson plans for the success of a clinician.

The supervisor needs lesson plans to guide and direct a clinician. The supervisor would be unable to encourage or discourage a clinician in the therapy performed without a lesson plan. The responsibilities of a supervisor rest on the fact that he knows what is going to happen before it happens. Without a lesson plan, the supervisor would be unaware of the objectives of the session and would be unable to recognize pitfalls before they occur. One prime responsibility of the supervisor is to assist the clinician in growing professionally. The problem without a lesson plan would be magnified because the clinician would need to do his altering after the mistakes were made which leads to much wasted therapy time. The supervisor could not make suggestions or modifications of the session, and the clinician would find himself in troublesome predicaments occasionally. The supervisor would be totally ineffective because there would be nothing to help him make his observations or evaluations except his subjective feelings. Then, personalities become the major factor of success or failure. The question might arise as to the intelligence or professional growth of a clinician, and without the written evidence, the lesson plan, there would be very little proof to the issue.

The client or the parents of the client expect some forward movement or some improvement in the speech of the client. It would seem to be a waste of time and money if progress was not made. Without a lesson plan, it would be difficult to determine if progress occurred. It would also be difficult to account for a lack of progress. When a lesson plan is used, it is easy to account to the parents or the client and explain that since this was tried and failed, then something new or different would have to be tried. It is, again, extremely difficult to know where success or failure exists without written evidence. The client is expected to perform certain tasks for the clinician. The clinician expects this performance. Then it only follows that an organized procedure must be followed in order to satisfy these expectations.

Thus the conclusion can be drawn that lesson plans are, indeed, necessary for the clinician, the supervisor, and the client. Lesson plans organize and direct the activities of all involved in the session.

### Why Are Lesson Plans Used?

Lesson plans are used in a variety of ways for a variety of reasons. Lesson plans are used to recognize strengths and weaknesses, to organize therapy sessions, to evaluate performance and development and to insure movement toward the established goals for the client.

The clinician uses the lesson plan to help him organize his plans. He establishes certain goals and by making a written note of the goals, he thinks them out. The clinician is encouraged to think things through. It is possible to make modifications in the established goals if they are well thought out in advance, but if they are not, then the task of modification is impossible. The clinician also uses the lesson plans as a guide for organizing the materials and supplies which are necessary for the days activities. Without lesson plans the clincian would waste valuable time in preparation and during actual therapy sessions. The student clinician is not knowledgeable, nor is he expected to be knowledgeable in every facet of therapy. That is why he is a student. He must seek help sometimes in planning the therapy sessions. By using the lesson plans, he recognizes his strengths and weaknesses. It is much easier for the student clinician to approach his supervisor and ask for help if he is able to indicate the specific area in which he is having problems.

The supervisor can locate strengths and weaknesses in the student clinician by careful study of his lesson plan. If the supervisor is alert, problems can be anticipated and encouragement given because of the lesson plan. A student clinician and the supervisor should have a working agreement whereby the student expects the supervisor to make suggestions prior to the therapy session based upon the objectives the student listed. Likewise, the supervisor should be prepared to help the student if need be. The supervisor, due to his responsible position, must recognize the appropriateness of an objective and the activity which will be used to reach the established goal. The supervisor should be acquainted with the situation and should allow the clinician to attempt new activities if they are well-thought out activities.

The primary purpose of the lesson plan for both clinician and supervisor is that of organization. If a lesson plan is not used, then the resulting session will not proceed smoothly. There will be much time wasted, and the preplanning sessions for subsequent sessions may become tedious. The rapport between clinician and supervisor may suffer as a result of poor planning and weak organization due to the absence of lesson plans.

## How Do You Write Lesson Plans?

Students, as well as practicing clinicians, should have long range goals as well as immediate goals. Clinicians are taught that terminal goals are a necessity. These goals describe the client's behavior that the clinician desires at the end of the therapy program. As the clinician describes the desired behavior, certain eventual goals become evident. The behavior which is desired cannot occur without planning. The unit plan or long range plan is composed of daily lesson plans which state specific goals or objectives and procedures that will be used to meet these objectives. Along with goals and procedures, the plans should include an evaluation of the day's procedures, and it should be noted whether success or failure resulted and why. If one waits too long, then the clinician and supervisor loose their objectivity.

Since the student clinician and supervisor use these plans to develop and organize, it must be remembered that the objectives must be measurable. A clinician cannot just write down what he wants to happen. The objective must be written in performance terms so that it specifies what the client must do or perform in order for him to reach the clinician's goals. In this way the clinician and the supervisor can observe the client and determine if the goal has or has not been met. An objective written, "To make Anne aware of the /r/ sound", is not enough. It should include a description of the behavior of the client. In this case no one knows what Anne will do to show that she is aware of the /r/ sound. The objective should be written, "To show that Anne is aware of the /r/ sound, she will be able to articulate accurately the /r/ sound while naming twenty-five pictures of objects containing the /r/ sound."

There are several reasons why lesson plans may be difficult to write. One of the first hurdles in developing a lesson plan is to answer three questions: the first is, "What is it I must teach?"; the second is, "What materials and procedures will work best to teach what it is I want to teach?"; and the third is, "How will I know when I have taught it?". If a clinician does not pay particular attention to writing objectives, he may find he cannot develop the lesson plan. It is rather difficult to find your way if you are not sure where you are going. It would be similar to the squirrel who wanted to seek his fortune. He put his material treasures in a little bundle, tied it onto a stick, put his few pennies into his pocket, kissed his mother and brothers and sisters goodbye, and began his search for fame and fortune. He had not been gone long when he came to a fork in the road. He was troubled as to which road to take--the one to the left or the one to the right. Suddenly a rabbit hopped by. He asked the squirrel, "Where are you going?"

"To seek my fame and fortune," replied the squirrel.

"Then you will need this," said the rabbit. And he showed the squirrel a rabbit's foot. "You will certainly need this for luck." "It will only cost you one of your treasures," added the rabbit. Gleefully the squirrel gave the rabbit the choice of one of his possessions. Both went away whistling gaily. Soon it began to get dark. The squirrel decided to look for a place to rest for the night. He sat down near a tree stump and presently he saw a fire-fly. He smiled and greeted the fire-fly. They began to talk. "Where are you going?" asked the fire-fly.

"To seek my fortune."

"Then you will need my light if you want to go on further," replied the fire-fly. "It will only cost you one of your treasures." So, eagerly, the squirrel purchased the light. He was certain he had the two things he needed to find his fortune, a rabbit's foot for luck and the fire-fly's light to show him the way.

He got up and continued on his way. It wasn't long until he saw a fox resting on a mailbox. After greeting each other, the fox asked, "Where are you going?"

"To find my fortune."

"Boy, you are in luck. Come with me and I'll show you the way." So they set off together, the squirrel and the fox. Soon the pair arrived at a house. "This is it," said the fox. He opened the door and the squirrel entered. That was the last anyone saw of the squirrel. But the fox looked pretty satisfied when he was last seen, and he remarked that squirrel stew had to be the greatest treat in the world.

The moral of this little fable is that without first establishing your specific destination, you may end up somewhere else.

It is not difficult to write behavioral objectives if one keeps in mind that they should be specific and measurable. An objective is meaningful if it communicates to the reader or supervisor the writer's intent. One thing that should be avoided if the objective is to be meaningful is the use of words or phrases which are open to many meanings or are ambiguous.

Consider the following words or phrases when determining the working of the behavorial objective:

| *Many Meanings* | *Few Meanings* |
| --- | --- |
| to appreciate | to compare and contrast |
| to believe | to build |
| to enjoy | to recite |
| to know | to produce |
| to understand | to differentiate |
| to have faith in | to identify |
| to understand fully | to say |
| to appreciate fully | to pronounce |

If a clinician uses words which are open to misunderstanding, he leaves himself in a rather vulnerable position. In order to avoid using these words or phrases with many meanings, the clinician should be very specific. If he finds it necessary to use words which are not explicit, then he should explain what he wants. For example: "The client will have faith in the clinician by selecting from a closed box the items he can correctly identify." This statemen has several words included which can cause misunderstandings. For example, faith is not explicit enough. Therefore, an explanation should accompany this objective. It should probably read: "The clinician will show the client pictures of items and the client will be able to receive miniature models of each item which he correctly identifies. The client will identify each item because he has faith that the client has a miniature model of every item in the closed box." In this way, the supervisor cannot misinterpret or misread the objective. Thus as the final evaluation is made, the proper interpretation is given. The question, "How can I write objectives which will describe specifically the desired response?" should be considered by both the clinician and the supervisor. It is difficult to prescribe concrete rules when one works with unique individuals. However, the following suggestions for writing behavioral objectives are usually more than satisfactory.

1. Specify the kind of behavior that will be accepted as proof that the client has satisfactorily reached the objective (*i.e.,* to recite, to pronounce, to compare.)

2. Identify the condition under which the behavior will occur (while the clinician shows him pictures, while looking at a familiar book, while listening to a recording).

3. Identify the limit of acceptable performance by describing how well the client must perform.

Again, these are merely guidelines. The clinician and supervisor must remember that the purpose of an objective is to communicate the intended outcome. Often times it is necessary to write several statements to describe the desired results. It is acceptable to write as many statements or objectives as are necessary in order to communicate the desired results. It should be stated here, however, that too many statements might indicate that too much is being attempted. It is extremely important that the daily lesson plans be narrowed down and not include more work than the client can comprehend. For successful lesson plans, much thought must be put into the amount to be included. The clinician must be realistic in what he desires the client to do. Each performance must be geared to the client. The client cannot be expected to perform tasks which are unrealistic. The conditions under which the performance is to be made should be familiar or explained so that the client is comfortable in the therapy setting. If in doubt as to the clarity of the objective, ask yourself, "Would it be possible for another clinician to use the objective to select successful learners?"

Once the objectives are written, and the clinician has determined what it is he is going to teach, he must then decide what materials and procedures are to be used to meet his goals. Just as in the  fable of the squirrel, a rabbit's foot for luck won't be sufficient nor will light. The clinician must find a way to use the materials so that they become useful tools. As was mentioned earlier in this chapter, the materials are gathered ahead of the therapy session, if at all possible.

Procedures determine the materials which are needed. The clinician should keep his procedures simple, keeping in mind the abilities of his client and the objectives he wrote guiding the session. The procedures should be well developed so the supervisor does not have to attempt to be clairvoyant. When one tries to read someone else's mind, misunderstandings often occur. Misunderstandings should be avoided whenever possible so that all persons involved in the clinical situation can have maximum success. Procedures should be written so that they follow in consecutive order. The order must be clear in the mind of the supervisor so he can give proper evaluation to the session; the procedure must be clear in the mind of the clinician so that clear instructions can be given to the client; and the procedures must be clear in the mind of the client so minimal amount of anxiety is experienced. If the client becomes frustrated due to the complexities of the procedures used in the session, negative results might occur.

If the procedures are not clearly established, the materials which are necessary cannot be prepared ahead of the therapy session. When a clinician is in a setting where supplies and materials are shared, it is a professional courtesy to plan ahead so that therapy sessions of other clinicians are not disturbed. It must be remembered that a clinician must have good rapport with other clinicians as well as his supervisor and client if he is to succeed in his clinical environment. A clinician must be able to accept the responsibility of preparing and maintaining supplies and materials. The supply cabinet or materials center must be kept neat and orderly if time and effort are to be saved for the therapy session. Often, if the clinician must search and dig for needed supplies and materials, an activity is forgotten or laid aside because the clinician does not have enough time to continue looking for the materials he needs. Had the materials been put away correctly, the activity could have been attempted. Just because a clinician is forgetful or irresponsible, the client may suffer. The novice clinician should spend several hours becoming acquainted with the supplies available to him. Often the clinician can get some good ideas for future activities by examining what materials are available to him. In most clinical settings, there is a limited budget and the clinician must learn to be resourceful and creative. Sometimes the simplest of activities can become a favorite of the client with a little effort and initiative by the clinician. The supervisor should encourage originality from the clinician and should not be tied to traditional procedures.

Evaluation of the session is of great importance to all. The clinician should evaluate as well as the supervisor. The clinician must evaluate immediately following the therapy session so there are no intervening distractions. The clinician is in the best position to evaluate critically the success or failure of a session. In order to make a proper evaluation of a therapy session, the clinician must ask himself several questions. First ask, "Did I follow my procedures carefully enough?" Second ask, "Was the client able to meet the objective satisfactorily?" To answer this question, the clinician must be able to specify if the client performed the necessary skills previously established. Also, the clinician cannot reduce his expectations. The objectives, if they were realistic, must be met exactly as they were stated. If the clinician notes that the client was able, let's say, to identify twenty kitchen items using /r/ as he examined the pictures of the items, yet the objective stated he should identify twenty-five, then this must be noted in the evaluation. The objective was not sufficiently reached, but maybe some progress was made, nevertheless. This will become more important as the new objectives for subsequent lesson plans are developed.

It is of utmost importance that the supervisor record his observations as he makes them. It is impossible to remember small, minute details after an intervening activity occurs. Progress or regression can be noted in the nonverbal or verbal activities which occur in the therapy room, and these activities may go unheeded or unnoticed by the clinician due to his involvement in the therapy session. It is the responsibility of the supervisor to note the activities and draw these to the attention of the clinician during the post-therapy session. Let it be noted here that the supervisor and clinician have a conference as soon after the observed therapy session as possible so that observations may be shared, activities modified, and anxieties removed. Anytime that a clinician is observed, certain anxieties are created. These must be calmed as soon as possible so that the clinician can function at maximum efficiency. Evaluations should be a time for constructive criticism rather than destructive criticism. A good rule for the supervisor to follow, as it is for anyone at anytime, is if you note something bad, try to balance that by noting something good. Remember a person likes to be told he had some successful activities; then the suggestions of ways to improve his shortcomings are more palatable. If the evaluation session is approached in a positive manner, then growth and progression will probably occur. Evaluations should be clearly stated and complete in important details so that they can serve as a useful basis for future lesson plans.

Table 1 represents a sample lesson plan form which might be used by the speech clinician. It can be noted that methods, procedures and materials are considered as one unit. If it is so desired by the supervisor, this section can be subdivided for clarity. In addition to the form, sample lesson plans are also included (Tables 2, 3, 4, and 5).

It is important that the information at the top of the page be included as it provides immediate reference for the supervisor. It is necessary that the supervisor who supervises many clinicians be familiar with each client so that proper criticism can be made.

TABLE 1
SAMPLE LESSON PLAN FORM
SPEECH AND HEARING CLINIC
University of North Dakota
WEEKLY LESSON PLAN

Client _____  Clinician _____  Date _____

Age _____  Immediate Supervisor _____  Hours of therapy
this semester _____

Disorder _____  Room and time _____

| Daily Objectives: (Itemize for each day) | Methods, Procedures and Materials: (Specify for each objective) | Evaluation: (Consider objectives, methods and materials, client progress and clinician effectiveness as appropriate) |
|---|---|---|
| | | |

**TABLE 2**
**SAMPLE LESSON PLAN**
SPEECH AND HEARING CLINIC
University of North Dakota
WEEKLY LESSON PLAN

| Client | John Smith | Clinician | Cheryl Ames | Date | February 17-20, 1977 |
|---|---|---|---|---|---|
| Age | 7 years, 8 months | Immediate Supervisor | Dr. Johnson | Hours of therapy this semester | 9½ |
| Disorder | Language/Articulation | Room and time | Blind School 11:00-11:30 a.m. | | |

| Daily Objectives: (Itemize for each day) | Methods, Procedures and Materials: (Specify for each objective) | Evaluation: (Consider objectives, methods and materials, client progress and clinician effectiveness as appropriate) |
|---|---|---|
| **Monday to Friday** 1. The client will receptively identify 10/10 pictures of clothing correctly. 2. The client will correctly respond in such behaviors as "push car." Verbs be used are: push, pull, touch. Nouns are: horse, car, baby carriage. 3. The client will produce 10/10 correct responses when asked to repeat the following sounds: /ma/, /mo/. 4. The client will produce 10/10 approximations of the following three words: comb, mine, car. **Friday** A one minute conversation sample will be taken and the number of identifiably correct words counted and charted. | 1. The client will be presented with two pictures and asked to identify the correct picture. Peabody cards and real clothing will be used. 2. The verbs will initially be trained on one noun, and understanding of the verbs will be tested by carryover to the other nouns. The client will initially imitate the clinician. 3. The client will imitate the clinician and correct phonetic placement will be emphasized. 4. Real objects and questions directed to the client will be used, e.g., "Whose is this?" "Mine." **Friday** Each correct response is reinforced 100% socially. Tokens are given for each correct response. An animal cracker is given to the client at the termination of each step (1-4) to encourage attending behavior. | 1. This goal was achieved. 2. The client identified "touch car" correctly but "push and pull car" only 6/10 times. 3. The client pulled his jaw back when pronouncing the initial consonant, so work was done on correct pronunciation of the /m/ sound. 4. The client produced /ko/ and /ka/ for comb and car but could not pronounce "mine" at all. **Friday** The one minute conversation sample revealed two identifiable words, the same as last week. Reinforcement appeared effective at the beginning of each session, but the client seemed disinterested during the last half of each session. The clinician should, perhaps, change reinforcers. |

TABLE 3
SAMPLE LESSON PLAN
SPEECH AND HEARING CLINIC
University of North Dakota
WEEKLY LESSON PLAN

Client ___John Smith___

Clinician ___Cheryl Ames___

Date ___February 9-13, 1977___

Age ___7 years, 8 months___

Immediate Supervisor ___Dr. Johnson___

Hours of therapy this semester ___7½___

Disorder ___Language/Articulation___

Room and time ___Blind School 11:0C-11:30 a.m.___

**Daily Objectives:**
(Itemize for each day)

**Monday to Friday**

1. The client will receptively identify 10/10 pictures of animals correctly.

2. The client will correctly respond in such behaviors as "push car." Verbs to be used are: push, pull, touch. Nouns are: horse, car, baby carriage.

3. The client will produce 10/10 correct responses when asked to repeat the following sounds /u/, /c/.

4. The client will produce 10/10 approximations of the following three words: ball, comb, key.

**Friday**
A one minute conversation sample will be taken and the number of identifiable correct words charted.

**Methods, Procedures and Materials:**
(Specify for each objective)

1. The client will be presented with 2 pictures and asked to point to the correct picture. Peabody pictures and story books with animals will be used.

2. The verbs will initially be trained on one noun, and understanding of the verbs will be tested by carryover to the other nouns. The client will initially imitate the clinician.

3. The client will imitate the clinician and will be reinforced for correct productions.

4. Real objects will be shown to the client, and he will be asked to identify them.

**Friday**
Each correct response is reinforced 100% socially. Tokens are given for each correct response. The client puts one token in a cup each time the clinician says "Good boy." An animal cracker is given to the client at the termination of each step (1, 2,3,4) to encourage attending behavior. These reinforcers appear to be the most effective thus far.

**Evaluation:**
(Consider objectives, methods and materials, client progress and clinician effectiveness as appropriate)

1. The client achieved this goal by the end of the week. His attention span for this was only good when this task was done at the beginning of the session.

2. The client correctly responded to "touch car," but confused "push and pull" 5/10 times, indicating poor discrimination between the two.

3. The client produced 10/10 correct responses here.

4. The client produced the following for the three words: /b/, /ko/, /ki/.

The one minute conversation sample revealed two identifiable words, an increase of two from last week.

The reinforcers were quite effective. However, the client has a very short attention span, so the activities should, perhaps, be shorter and changed often.

**TABLE 4**
**SAMPLE LESSON PLAN**
SPEECH AND HEARING CLINIC
University of North Dakota

**WEEKLY LESSON PLAN**

| | | |
|---|---|---|
| Client    Dennis Olson | Clinician    Kathy Jones | Date   February 17-20, 1977 |
| Age    8 years | Immediate Supervisor    Dr. Johnson | Hours of therapy |
| Disorder    Language/Articulation | Room and time    Blind School 10:30-11:00 a.m. | this semester    9½ |

**Daily Objectives:**
(Itemize for each day)

**Monday to Friday**

**Semantics**
1. The client will identify 15 pictures of clothing both receptively and expressively.
2. The client will correctly identify the following singular and plurals: man, men; tooth, teeth; foot, feet.

**Syntax**
1. The client will produce 10 sentences of the following pattern to teach the "not" concept:

He
She + is + not + verb + ing
It

**Phonology**
1. The client will produce 10/10 correct /f/ sounds in isolation and in syllables.
2. The client will produce 10/10 correct /f/ sounds in words, initial position.

**Friday**
A one minute conversation sample will be taken and the number of correctly produced words will be counted and charted.

**Methods, Procedures and Materials:**
(Specify for each objective)

**Semantics**
1. Initially, the client will be shown 2 Peabody cards and will be asked to point to the correct one, after which the client will be asked to identify clothing expressively. Real clothing will also be used, as well as the Peabody Mannequin dolls.
2. The real objects and pictures will be used and the client will be asked to respond appropriately.

**Syntax**
1. Situation pictures will be used. The client will respond to questions asked by the clinician, such as: "Is he jumping?" The client will respond, "He is not jumping." Imitation will be used initially.

**Phonology**
1. Correct phonetic placement will be emphasized.
2. Pictures of words beginning with /f/ will be used.

**Friday**
Social reinforcement will be emphasized. If the client produces enough responses to fill a cup with tokens, he will be able to paste a sticker in a sticker book and on Fridays will receive gum.

**Evaluation:**
(Consider objectives, methods and materials, client progress and clinician effectiveness as appropriate)

**Semantics**
The client achieved this goal by the end of the week. The methods used were effective.

The client correctly identified the plurals, but not the singulars by the end of the week.

**Syntax**
The client had great difficulty here. Imitation was used all week, only repeating the last 2 elements of the sentence, e.g., not swimming. It appears that the client cannot remember the sentence when imitating the clinician.

**Phonology**
10/10 correct /f/ sounds in isolation, 8/10 correct /f/ sounds in syllables was achieved.

This goal was not attempted since the client did not reach 10/10 correct /f/ sounds in syllables.

Conversation sample revealed 10 correctly produced words per minute. (An increase of one from last week.)

**Friday**
Reinforcement appeared to be extremely effective.

TABLE 5
SAMPLE LESSON PLAN
SPEECH AND HEARING CLINIC
University of North Dakota
WEEKLY LESSON PLAN

Client ___Dennis Olson___  Clinician ___Kathy Jones___  Date March 1-5, 1977

Age ___8 years___  Immediate Supervisor ___Dr. Johnson___  Hours of therapy ___13½___ this semester

Disorder ___Language/Articulation___  Room and time  Blind School  10:30-11:00 a.m.

**Daily Objectives**
(Itemize for each day)

**Monday to Friday**

**Semantics**
1. The client will identify pictures of transportation vehicles both receptively and expressively.
2. The client will correctly identify the following irregular singular and plurals: Man, men; Tooth, teeth; foot, feet.

**Syntax**
1. The client will produce 10 sentences of the following pattern to teach the "not" concept:

He
She + is + not + verb + ing
It

**Phonology**
1. The client will produce 10/10 correct /f/ sounds in isolation, and in syllables.

**Friday**
A one minute conversation sample will be taken and the number of correctly produced words will be counted and charted.

**Methods, Procedures and Materials:**
(Specify for each objective)

**Semantics**
1. Peabody pictures will be presented to the client and he will be asked to tell what they are.
2. Real objects and pictures will be used.

**Syntax**
1. Situation pictures and verb cards will be used. The client will respond to the question, "Is he sleeping" with the response, "He is not sleeping." Imitation will be used initially.

**Phonology**
1. Correct phonetic placement and direction of the airflow will be emphasized.

**Friday**
Social reinforcement will be emphasized. If the client produces enough responses to fill a cup with tokens, he will be able to paste a sticker in a sticker book and on Fridays will receive gum.

**Evaluation:**
(Consider objectives, methods and materials, client progress and clinician effectiveness as appropriate)

**Semantics**
1. The client achieved this goal by the end of the week.
2. The client correctly identified all of these by the end of the week. However, he occasionally gave the plural for the singular when not concentrating.

**Syntax**
1. The client correctly imitated the clinician when repeating not + verb + ing.

**Phonology**
1. The client produced close approximations of the /f/ sound in isolation. It appeared to be too breathy. Closer approximations will be demanded of him. The client did, however, produce 9/10 correct /f/ syllables.

**Friday**
The one minute conversation sample revealed 12 correctly pronounced words, and increase of one from last week. Reinforcement was quite effective.

## Summary

The lesson plan was discussed in some detail. The questions what is a lesson plan, who needs a lesson plan, why is a lesson plan used, and how do you write a lesson plan were answered.

The lesson plan is a guide for both clinician and supervisor. It serves to organize the therapy session so that all participants in the session, the clinician, the supervisor, and the client, can have maximum success. If lesson plans are not developed for the entire unit and for daily sessions, needless time will be lost. The sessions will be unsuccessful, the clinician and client will be frustrated, and the supervisor will not be able to fulfill her responsibilities to the development of a trained clinician.

The lesson plan is a necessary tool to the therapy session. Without it, the clinician would have no way of knowing where to advance with the therapy of a client, no idea of what to do in order to help the client, and least of all, the clinician would have no activities or plans in mind for the client. Goals must be established and plans must evolve around these goals so that success may be achieved. Not all goals will be reached, but lesson plans will also allow evaluations to be made which should assist both clinician and supervisor.

Lesson plans should contain behavioral objectives, procedures, materials and supplies for the planned activities and evaluations. Since the lesson plans are used to develop and organize the therapy session, the objectives should be written so they are measurable. Words which have many definitions or are ambiguous should be avoided and words which are specific in meaning should be used in writing the behavioral objectives. Suggestions for the writing of behavioral objectives are: 1) specify the behavior, 2) identify the conditions, and 3) identify the limit of acceptable performance. Once the objectives are written, then activities should be chosen which will help the clinician reach the established goals. Materials should be organized ahead of the established therapy session so that minimal time is spent in getting prepared for the session as therapy begins. Once the therapy session ends, both clinician and supervisor should evaluate the session so that proper criticisms can be made. A sample lesson plan for this is suggested. It includes some necessary information which will be useful to the supervisor.

If lesson plans are approached with a positive attitude, they can be both profitable and helpful.

## Questions and Issues

1. How important is it to the novice student clinicians to develop appropriate lesson plans? How important is it for the experienced clinician to develop appropriate lesson plans?

2. The organization of a lesson plan is unimportant as long as the lesson plan contains the appropriate procedures and objectives. Take a position regarding this statement and support it.

3. Learning to create good lesson plans is usually learned quickly and with minimal effort. Take a position regarding this statement and support it.

4. What is the value of writing evaluations of procedures and objectives stated on the lesson plan soon after the therapy session?

5. Is it meaningful to store lesson plans for future use and reference? Explain your answer.

# CHAPTER 3

## OBSERVATION EVALUATION SYSTEMS

### Introduction and Background

Interaction analysis is a technique whereby events which occur between two or more people can be identified and studied. An event is the specific behavior which occurs within a specified time and is recorded by an observer using a coded system.

The purposes of interaction analysis are to study, control, and change behavior. This is accomplished by transcribing selected behavioral events, thus providing a means of identifying behaviors under examination. From the attained information, behaviors can be modified.

Interaction analysis or, commonly termed, observation systems are used in various professions. They are used in universities where student teachers are trained, in specific areas of education where improvement of teaching performance is a goal, in industry and business, in medical training institutions, in psychotherapy, and in clinical situations where specific therapy is administered. Numerous observation instruments which are referred to as category systems are in use today. Presently, Simon and Boyer (1967) cite approximately seventy-eight observation instruments.

A number of educational institutions involved in teacher training employ interaction analysis as a tool in the training process. The student teachers use the interaction analysis to gain information so they may learn to control their behavior in the classroom. Most of the systems used for observation are based upon the Flanders' Interaction Analysis Categories which were developed by Flanders at the University of Minnesota between 1955-1960 (1970).

This interaction analysis system, commonly called the Flanders' System, employs ten categories. Seven categories are used when the teacher is talking. They are: Accepts Feelings, Praises or Encourages, Accepts or Uses Ideas of Pupils, Asks Questions, Lectures or Gives Direction, and Criticizes or Justifies Authority. The two categories used when the pupil is talking are Pupil-Talk-Response and Pupil-Talk-Initiation. The last category is Silence or Confusion. Flanders (1970) states that the use of these ten categories exhausts all possible events which can take place in the classroom.

The Flanders' System is used by having an observer sit in the classroom and record a behavior every three seconds by writing a number from the category system which identifies what the teacher or the class is doing. The observer must have memorized the coded numbers which represent the behavior to record the classroom action accurately.

The original purpose of the Flanders' Interaction Analysis Categories System was to analyze the initiatory and response behavior characteristics between two or more individuals. With this system, an estimate of the balance of time between initiative and response behaviors can be inferred by comparing the percentage of time the teacher talks, the pupil talks, and the silence and confusion. The percentage of time contributed to each of the ten behavioral categories can also be calculated.

The Flanders' Categories have been widely used in a variety of teaching situations and teacher training activities to provide teachers with feedback about their own teaching behaviors and the quantity of student participation in their classrooms.

Several systems have been adapted from the Flanders' System because of the desire for additional information. The Flanders' Expanded System was developed by Flanders (1967) and was built upon the ten categories of the original instrument by dividing eight of the categories for more discrete recording of observed behaviors. The category entitled Praises or Encourages (Category 2) was expanded to discriminate between "superficial" versus more "genuine" praise; the category called Giving Directions, Commands, or Orders (Category 6) was broadened to reflect differences between demands for "unquestioning obedience" versus commands which "allow for alternative proposals". Another category which was expanded was Silence (Category 10) which was divided into "non-constructive" versus "constructive" use of time.

Amidon and Hunter (1966) have expanded the Flanders' System into what they call the Verbal Interaction Category System (VICS). This system included not only the teacher's acceptance or rejection of the students' verbal behavior, but also measured the non-verbal behavior of the teacher and student. These authors have also separated "Silence" from "Confusion" in their system. In addition, the VICS reveals the physical freedom of the pupil.

An observation system developed by Aschner and Gallagher, the Aschner-Gallagher System (1967), focuses on the thought processes in the classroom. This is a complex system with five major categories and forty-seven subcategories.

One observation system which was designed to chart the stage of development of any group in various phases of problem solving is the Sequential Analysis of Verbal Interaction (SAVI) developed by Simon and Agazarian (1967). This system contains nine classes of verbal behavior expressed by twenty-eight major categories. It can be used effectively, however, with as few as four of the categories. The SAVI was designed for use in a variety of settings, and, since it is not necessary to use all of the categories at any one time, it has flexibility which increases its usefulness.

Another system described by Amidon and Hunter (1966) is the Modified Category System (MCS). This system was developed at Temple University by the College of Education staff interested in improving teaching skills. Observation systems such as the Aschner-Gallagher, Medley, Hugher-Miller, and Simon and Agazaran were reviewed by the staff. The education staff members proceeded to integrate what they felt were the best parts of each reviewed system into the Flanders' System. Thus, a new system was derived which added a new dimension to observation systems. When using the MCS, an observer moved from student to student coding the first, unambiguous behavior observed for each student. A typical round took two or three minutes, and twelve to twenty-four rounds constituted a sample.

Several educational areas have developed observation systems which are adapted to a specific area of the curriculum. For example, Moskowitz (1967) designed the Foreign Language Inter-action System (FLint) which is a direct outgrowth of the Flanders' System of Interaction Analysis. The FLint System focuses on behavior commonly used in the classroom where students are taught foreign language. It identifies whether the foreign language or the native tongue is being spoken and identifies such elements as direct pattern drills or repetition of students' words.

The Oliver-Shaver System, discussed by Oliver and Shaver (1962) was developed to determine the teaching style of those teachers dealing with controversial issues in social studies classes. This study focuses on the basis for statements causing intense emotional involvement.

Observation systems which have been developed in other areas of the curriculum include the Wright System (Wright, 1967), mathematics; Science Observation System (Altman, 1970), science; Parakh Pupil Verbal-Behavior Category System (Parakh, 1967), biology; and Modes of Communication (Roberts, 1968), religious education.

Another type of observation system is the Instrument for the Observation of Teaching Activities called IOTA which was developed by the National IOTA Council. This differs from the system described earlier in that it involves a written description of class-room behavior by a team of at least three observers who are familiar with the system. It also utilizes an interview with the teacher at a time other than the observation period. The IOTA is concerned with the teacher's role, rather than with the interaction process. Six areas of teacher competence, as stated in *Role of the*

*Teacher in Society* National IOTA Council, 1970), form the basis of this instrument. These areas are: 1) Director of learning, 2) Counselor and advisor, 3) Mediator of the culture, 4) Link with the community, 5) Member of the staff and 6) Member of the teaching profession.

The IOTA also includes a set of criteria for twenty-seven teaching acts based on the six areas of teacher competence. These teaching acts are divided into two sections, fourteen behavioral acts which are identified during the observation session, and thirteen behavioral acts which are verified by the teacher at the time of the interview. Through observation and interview sessions, it is possible to develop a profile of a teacher's performance.

The IOTA focuses on objectivity, not subjectivity, and is specific rather than general. The teacher is not compared with another teacher at any time, but is measured against accepted criteria established by the National IOTA Council.

"IOTA is an instrument for the evaluation of teaching competence and is to be used only for the improvement of instruction" (Deever, Demeke, and Wochner, 1971). The IOTA is weighted toward self-analysis and self-evaluation leading to self-improvement.

The IOTA has been adapted for observations in the field of speech and hearing, and it has been used with clinicians in the public school systems. The twenty-seven categories were modified to be applicable to therapy situations rather than to the classroom. The observation and interview session procedures remained unchanged, and they resulted in a profile of clinical behaviors for each clinician.

Even though the IOTA has been used to examine teacher activities, observation systems are more commonly used. Some of the divisions of education which have used interaction analysis are: special education, Hill Interaction Matrix (Hill, 1965); curriculum development, System for Analyzing Lessons (Herbert, 1967) and Clements System (Clements, 1967); social work, Moustakas-Siegel-

Schalock System (Moustakas, Sigel, and Schalock, 1955) and Family Interaction System (Riskin, 1964); and guidance and Counseling, Resource Processing Coding System (Longabaugh, 1969).

In professions other than education, observation systems are used to measure such areas as personnel management, integration in industry, decision making, and small group situations where tensions exist.

The Argyris System (1966) focuses on dimensions of inter-personal competence in industrial settings. The groups being observed can vary in size from as few as two to as many as fifty individuals. The length of observation time varies, also. Usually this system is used at meetings where the members of the group are concerned with problem-solving. Therefore, some meetings are longer than others, but the total time of the observation is usually fifty-five to sixty minutes. Some of the categories measured are: 1) Does the member help others? 2) Does the member have concern for others? 3) Is the member antagonistic? 4) Does the member mistrust the others? and 5) Does the member have original ideas?

In addition to the Argyris System, additional interaction analysis systems exist which have been designed to assist in analyz-ing professional behaviors. The Sequential Analysis of Verbal Interaction (Simon and Agazarian, 1967) and the Melbin System (Melbin, 1954) have also been used in business and industrial set-tings. The A. Anderson System (Anderson, 1966) and the Medical Instruction Observation Record (Jason, 1962), are applied in the fields of medicine and dentistry; whereas, psychologists have employed the Snyder System (Snyder and June, 1961).

Although education has received major emphasis for research-ers in the development of observational systems, other areas have also profited from these systems which serve as a means of identi-fying behaviors, analyzing patterns of conduct, and encouraging desired changes.

## The ABC System: Introduction

The first evidence of the use of an interaction analysis system for observation and supervision of clinical practicum in speech pathology appeared in 1970. The Boone-Prescott 10 Category System (Boone and Steck, 1970; and Boone and Prescott, 1970) provided a method for analyzing clinical behaviors using self-evaluation. Boone and Prescott's system which consists of ten categories is based upon learning theory. This system allows the clinician to qualify his behavior for self-evaluation. The first five categories relate to clinician activities and last five to client behavior. The system and scoring procedures can be found in Boone and Prescott (1972b).

Schubert and Miner (1970), who were unaware of the Boone-Prescott 10 Category System, were developing an observation system at approximately the same time. The Schubert-Miner system was derived directly from the original Flanders' system (Flanders, 1967). Schubert and Miner originally titled their observation system the Modification of Flanders' Interaction Analysis Categories for Observation in Speech Therapy. The categories of clinical behavior as they appeared in the original system are presented in Table 6. The system includes twelve categories, eight pertaining to clinician behavior, two to client behavior, and the last two categories applied to both client and clinician behavior.

The Schubert and Miner system was developed to quantify the behaviors observed during the therapy session, and to enable the supervisor and student clinician to recall and analyze the behaviors and sequential patterns which occurred. Clinician-client behaviors are recorded at three second intervals by writing the numbers corresponding to the behavior occurring at that time.

The important differences between the Schubert-Miner and the Boone-Prescott systems are as follows:

| Boone-Prescott System | Schubert-Miner System |
|---|---|
| Total of ten categories<br>five categories centering on client behavior<br><br>five categories centering on clinician behavior | Total of twelve categories<br>two categories centering on client behavior<br><br>eight categories centering on clinician behavior<br><br>two categories pertaining to client and/or client-clinician behavior |
| Recording is determined by change in behavioral pattern | Recording is determined by time. A number relating to the occurring clinician-client behavior is recorded every three seconds |
| Based on learning theory | Based on the Flanders' Interaction Analysis System and clinician-client behavior observed by the supervisor of clinical practicum |
| Behavior is video-taped and analyzed at a later time | Behavior is recorded live and analyzed immediately |

**TABLE 6**
**MODIFICATION OF FLANDERS' INTERACTION**
**ANALYSIS CATEGORIES FOR OBSERVATION**
**IN SPEECH THERAPY**

| | |
|---|---|
| **THERAPIST TALK** | 1. **ACCEPTS CLIENT'S RESPONSE AND USES IT:** developing and using response or action of the client. |
| | 2. **INSTRUCTION AND DEMONSTRATION :** process of giving verbal instruction or showing the client procedures to be used. Explain how something is to be done. |
| | 3. **AUDIO—STIMULATION AND QUESTIONS:** intent that the client will respond. |
| | 4. **VISUAL STIMULATION AND QUESTIONS:** intent that the client will respond. |
| | 5. **AUDIO AND/OR VISUAL REINFORCEMENT OF CLIENT'S CORRECT RESPONSE.** |
| | 6. **RELATING USELESS INFORMATION AND ASKING IMPERTINENT QUESTIONS.** |
| | 7. **CRITICIZING OR USING AUTHORITY:** action used to change behavior from an unacceptable to an acceptable pattern. |
| | 8. **REINFORCEMENT OF INCORRECT RESPONSE.** |
| **CLIENT TALK** | 9. **CLIENT'S RESPONSE:** client response to direct stimulus of the therapist. Attempts to respond to a stimulus initiating change in speech pattern. |
| | 10. **CLIENT'S RESPONSE:** talking and responding in a manner unrelated to changing speech pattern. |
| | 11. **SILENCE** |
| | 12. **CONFUSION :** disorder in which communication cannot be understood or observed. |

## TABLE 7
## ANALYSIS OF BEHAVIOR OF CLINICIANS (ABC) SYSTEM

| | Category | Definition |
|---|---|---|
| **CLINICIAN BEHAVIOR** | 1. Observing and Modifying Lesson Appropriately | Using response or action of the client to adjust goals and/or strategies |
| | 2. Instruction and Demonstration | Process of giving instruction or demonstrating the procedures to be used |
| | 3. Auditory and/or Visual Stimulation | Questions, cues, and models intended to elicit a response |
| | 4. Auditory and/or Visual Positive Reinforcement of Client's Correct Response | Process of giving any positive response to correct client response |
| | 5. Auditory and/or Visual Negative Reinforcement of Client's Incorrect Response | Process of giving any negative response to an incorrect client response |
| | 6. Auditory and/or Visual Positive Reinforcement of Client's Incorrect Response | Process of giving any positive response to an incorrect client response |
| | 7. Clinician Relating Irrelevant Information and/or Asking Irrelevant Questions | Talking and/or responding in a manner unrelated to changing speech patterns |
| | 8. Using Authority or Demonstrating Disapproval | Changing social behavior from unacceptable to acceptable behavior |
| **CLIENT BEHAVIOR** | 9. Client Responds Correctly | Client responds appropriately, meets expected level |
| | 10. Client Responds Incorrectly | Client apparently tries to respond appropriately but response is below expected level |
| | 11. Client Relating Irrelevant Information and/or Asking Irrelevant Questions | Talking and/or responding in a manner unrelated to changing speech patterns |
| | 12. Silence | Absence of verbal and relevant motor behavior |

Boone, Miner and Schubert are in agreement that the use of an interaction analysis system is a valuable tool in creating behavioral changes in student clinicians. Observation systems also provide an objective means of quantifying and analyzing clinical behavior.

## Development of the ABC System

The Analysis of Behaviors of Clinicians (ABC) System is the final product of what was first called the Modification of Flanders' Interaction Analysis Categories for Observation in Speech Pathology.

A study was conducted in 1971 to study the usefulness of the original Interaction Analysis System. Clinical supervisors were asked to use the system; then they were asked to comment and make suggestions. From these suggestions the Analysis of Behaviors of Clinicians System was devised as shown in Table 7.

Category number 12, Confusion, from the Modified Flanders' System was omitted when structuring the ABC System. Early examination of the Modified Flanders' System clearly demonstrated this category to be useless. Category number 3, audio stimulation and category number 4, visual stimulation from the Modified Flanders' system were found not to be readily observable as separate categories. As a result, the two categories were combined in the ABC System, and they appear as category 4, Auditory or Visual stimulation.

A new category was listed as category 5, Negative Reinforcement of the Client's Incorrect Response. Negative reinforcement is defined as the clinician informing the client that his response to the stimulus was incorrect. The behavior was added because it was noted by personnel involved in the pilot study as occurring with noticeable regularity and no category existed for recording this behavior. It was concluded that this behavior was important and needed to be identified.

A second new category on the ABC System was number 10, Client Responds Incorrectly. Clinical supervisors involved in the pilot study were in agreement that the knowledge of this client behavior was important when examining the success of the expected goals established by the clinician. By recording this behavior, clinicians and supervisors have a more precise transcription of the therapy session. It was deemed important that clinicians and supervisors be aware of the correct and incorrect response ratios of the client as well as the clinician's reaction to this client behavior.

On both systems, the first eight categories pertained to the clinical behaviors of the clinician. The ABC System has three categories serving to record client behaviors; whereas, the Modified Flanders' System has two categories in this area. The ABC System has one clinician-client category, Silence. The Modified Flanders' had two categories, number 11, Silence, and number 12, Confusion. The ABC System includes eleven of the twelve behavioral categories used in the pilot study, plus two new behavioral categories. Consequently, the ABC System consists of twelve behavioral categories, eleven of which appeared on the Modified Flanders' System, one category, Confusion, was discarded, two categories were combined, and two categories were added.

Nine of the original behaviors appeared useful and remained essentially unchanged on the ABC System with slight terminology changes for purposes of clarification: Observing and Modifying Behavior, Giving Instructions and Demonstration, Reinforcing Client's Correct Response, Clinician Relating Irrelevant Information, Clinician Using Authority, Clinician Reinforcing Incorrect Response, Client Responding Correctly, Client Relating Irrelevant Information, and Silence.

Renumbering the categories 5, 6, 7, 8, 10 and 11 provided for better grouping and ease of memorization. Other changes included omitting or combining categories and adding new categories to the system.

The final minor revision regarding the Analysis of Behavior of Clinicians System occurred in 1974. To clarify category 5, the name of the category was changed from Auditory and/or Visual Negative Reinforcement of Client's Incorrect Response to that of Punishment.

## The ABC System: Purpose

The purpose of the Analysis of Behavior of Clinicians (ABC) System is to provide a means of recording clinician-client behaviors so that the behaviors can be quantified, analyzed, and, when appropriate, changed. The ABC System provides a method for the clinician and/or supervisor to record objectively what is occurring during a therapy session for immediate analysis or analysis at a later time.

From the analyzed data, the clinician and/or supervisor can make or set definite goals in relationship to future changes desired during the therapy session. Again, by using the ABC System of recording and analyzing data, it is possible to determine if the goals have been met or if there has been movement in the desired or recommended direction.

## The ABC System: Description

During a typical speech or language therapy session, interaction between the clinician and the client is the essential element one observes as a clinician seeks to elicit a given response from a client, and rewards him for his correct response or acceptable attempts and punishes him for incorrect response or unacceptable attempts. At times, observers note that the therapy session is heavily weighted with clinician behavior as the clinician attempts to explain, demonstrate, instruct, establish a friendly social relationship, or lavish praise on the client. Other therapy sessions are composed primarily of client response with the clinician in the background, serving as a listener, a stimulator, or an agent for change. The author of the ABC Category System has identified twelve behaviors based upon earlier research by Flanders and Boone and on two pilot studies conducted at the University of North Dakota and the University of Washington. These categories are not purported to be all inclusive, but they do represent some important segments of clinician-client behavior observed in typical therapy sessions.

The Analysis of Behavior of Clinicians (ABC) System is a twelve category time-based behavior recording system. By employing this system, a particular behavioral event can be placed into one of the twelve categories. The first eight categories describe the actions of the clinician as he attempts to elicit a response from the client, utilize rewards, modify his procedures in terms of the client's response, use authority, or as he fails to attend to the therapy task. The behavioral categories listed as nine through eleven indicate the action of the client as he responds correctly or incorrectly to the clinician and his attempts to avoid responding by irrelevant statements or questions. The final category, number twelve, Silence, occurs when both the clinician and the client display no verbal or relevant motor behavior. The categories and a brief description of each category are presented in Table 8.

It is important to become thoroughly familiar with each category and to identify a number of clinician or client acts that might be classified under each category before attempting to observe and to record the various behaviors. When using this system, behaviors are recorded at three second intervals. Following are the twelve categories and a discussion of each.

## The ABC System: Discussion of Categories

*Category 1:* Clinician observes the client and modifies lesson appropriately.

The ability to plan a therapy session has long been considered a desirable skill on the part of clinicians, but a skill placed somewhat higher on the hierarchy of clinical abilities is that identified as category one. It indicates that the clinician has been able to modify the planned action, change a goal, or alter a strategy in terms of the response the client makes to the stimulus. For example, the clinician may ask a child to produce a target phoneme in a nonsense syllable, but in response to the request the client says a word with the target phoneme uttered correctly. The

**TABLE 8**
**ANALYSIS OF BEHAVIOR OF CLINICIANS (ABC) SYSTEM,**
Revised 1974

| | | |
|---|---|---|
| **CLINICIAN BEHAVIOR** | 1. Observing and Modifying Lesson Appropriately | Using response or action of the client to adjust goals and/or strategies |
| | 2. Instruction and Demonstration | Process of giving instruction or demonstrating the procedures to be used |
| | 3. Auditory and/or Visual Stimulation | Questions, cues, and models intended to elicit a response |
| | 4. Auditory and/or Visual Positive Reinforcement of Client's Correct Response | Process of giving any positive response to correct client response |
| | 5. Punishment | Process of giving any negative response to an incorrect client response |
| | 6. Auditory and/or Visual Positive Reinforcement of Client's Incorrect Response | Process of giving any positive response to an incorrect client response |
| | 7. Clinician Relating Irrelevant Information and/or Asking Irrelevant Questions | Talking and/or responding in a manner unrelated to changing speech patterns |
| | 8. Using Authority or Demonstrating Disapproval | Changing social behavior from unacceptable to acceptable behavior |
| **CLIENT BEHAVIOR** | 9. Client Responds Correctly | Client responds appropriately, meets expected level |
| | 10. Client Responds Incorrectly | Client apparently tries to respond appropriately but response is below expected level |
| | 11. Client Relating Irrelevant Information and/or Asking Irrelevant Questions | Talking and/or responding in a manner unrelated to changing speech patterns |
| | 12. Silence | Absence of verbal and relevant motor behavior |

clinician may immediately change the request from one of repeating a nonsense syllable to one of correctly producing the target phoneme in this word or other words. Another example occurs when a clinician gives a model "carrying phrase" and asks the child to use it; but the client changes the "carrying phrase" to one which is easier for him, and the clinician utilizes the child's phrase rather than insisting on the one used as a model. The modification of a demand, and the alteration of the therapy session occurs when the response is better than the clinician expected, or it is not as good, or is different, and suggests another approach to the goal. It is easier to recognize a category one behavior when the lesson plans are available or the goal is known, but this is not always essential. This category is an unplanned response of the clinician to the client's behavior.

*Category 2:* Clinician instructs and/or demonstrates.

The processes of giving directions, explaining a procedure, showing precisely how a speech or communication activity is to be conducted, or describing a motor act are all important aspects of the therapy session. There are many approaches used by clinicians to get the client to perform the desired speech or language behavior. Games, toys, books, role playing, sentence building, discussions, utilization of mechanical devices such as the tape recorders or language masters, or demonstration in front of a mirror may be important therapy strategies. The clinician's behavior in giving directions, offering explanations, or demonstrating how to perform an act required of the client all come within this category. The explanation of a game, the instruction to "come to the mirror with your chair and I will show you how to place your lips for the /s/ sound" are common examples. The extent to which category two is used will depend, to a large extent, on the clinician's ability to simplify directions, and to give pertinent, meaningful demonstrations.

*Category 3:* The clinician provides auditory and/or visual stimulation.

This clinical procedure is thought to be a more specific one than the category just described. Category three indicates that the clinician has presented the exact word or sound or sentence to the client who is expected to repeat it as: Clinician: "Say what I say: Soon." Client: "Soon." The stimulation may be a visual one in which the clinician shows a picture or presents reading matter and expects the client to say the word without any auditory clue. A frequently used visual stimuli is the "number cue" used to show how many times the client is to repeat the correct phoneme, word, or sentence without interruption from the clinician. The observer will note that the stimuli may be auditory, visual, or a combination of the two, but the intent is that the client's response will be forthcoming with little or no delay.

*Category 4:* The clinician provides auditory and/or visual positive reinforcement of the client's correct response.

If a client responds correctly, the clinician often provides some type of positive reinforcement to encourage a repetition of the correct response either at the next response, or at some future time. Reinforcers take a variety of forms such as the verbal, "That's right!"; "Good talking!"; "Good! Say it again!"; or the nonverbal gesture indicating "Repeat what you just did," the smile or nod of approval, use of a counting device, or a primary reinforcer such as food. Occasionally, the reinforcer is a social one in which the clinician listens to the client and carries out a command or request, or carries on a conversation, or does not interrupt as long as the speech or language response is satisfactory. The positive reinforcer may be used on a regular reinforcement schedule if such a schedule is a planned part of the therapy program, or it may be used at irregular intervals depending on the needs of the client and the philosophy of the clinician. As used in category four, the positive reinforcer always follows a correct response of the client.

*Category 5:* Punishment

When the client responds incorrectly, the clinician has several choices of behavior. One choice is to indicate in some way that the response was not correct. This may be in the form of words such as, "No, that's not right!"; "Try again!"; "That's your old sound!"; "Did that sound right?"; or it may be a frown, a shake of the head, a gesture with thumbs down, or any signal known to mean the response was not correct. Punishment is less common than positive reinforcement; however, it may be necessary to provide both punishment and positive reinforcement to help the client perceive the difference between this correct and incorrect response pattern. A category five behavior (punishment) has the intent of letting the client know that his attempt was incorrect.

*Category 6:* The clinician provides auditory and/or visual positive reinforcement of the client's incorrect response.

As had been indicated earlier, an incorrect response offers the clinician a choice of several behaviors, one is to provide a positive reinforcer. This behavior normally occurs when the clinician is, in some way, unaware that the response was incorrect, or when he is so desirous of having the client continue his efforts that he reinforces with an indication that the response was correct even though it was not. The verbal and non-verbal reinforcers are the same as those described under category four, but in this instance they follow an incorrect attempt on the part of the client to perform as directed by the clinician. The most common examples are those which take place in articulation therapy when a client does not adequately produce a target phoneme, but the clinician rewards any attempt as though it were the desired one. As used in category six, the positive reinforcer always follows an incorrect response.

*Category 7:* Clinician relates useless information and/or asks irrelevant questions.

This category indicates that the clinician's behavior is not directed toward securing a response from the client, nor in any way rewarding his attempts to respond. Earlier recording with this category indicated that clinicians may spend considerable time during the therapy session carrying on a conversation with the client or relating some kind of information which is not goal directed. In most instances, this type of behavior seems to have little or no usefulness, but it is occasionally used in an effort to "establish rapport," "gain insight into the client's problem," or for some other stated purpose. When the purpose is one of establishing or maintaining a friendly client-clinician relationship, or of providing a momentary period of much needed relaxation, the observer is usually quickly aware of the purpose and may, indeed, score such behavior as a category one. However, when a continuous period of unnecessary conversation between the clinician and client or an extended period of "chattering" by the clinician takes place, the behavior is obviously contributing little or nothing to the therapy session and should be regarded as a category seven.

*Category 8:* The clinician uses authority and/or demonstrates disapproval of client's behavior.

This category is usually used in relationship to the client's social behavior and is more frequently observed in the therapy situation with younger children than with adults. It usually occurs when the clinician is aware that the client is attempting to avoid the therapy task whether or not it is a difficult one for him to perform. The category is not meant to suggest that this is negative behavior on the part of the clinician; it merely implies that the clinician recognizes the client's evasive or avoidance behavior and is attempting to deal with it in a direct way. Common examples are noted when the clinician says such things as: "Let's get busy and see how quickly you can complete this." "Sit up in your chair and show me how hard you can work for five minutes." "John, we do not bother other people in this school."; "We can't wait for you any longer; now it is＿＿＿＿＿＿＿'s turn." The behavior may be nonverbal when the clinician frowns, shakes his head, points to a specific chair, crayon, or indicates a task previously requested of the child. The change in vocal tone, rate of speaking, or in carefully controlled wording is sometimes an indication that the clinician is using authority as a means of control, and may reflect knowledge that the particular client responds best to this pattern, or may be a reflection of the clinician's tolerance level. Regardless of the cause or of the positive or negative effect of the authoritative behavior, all such actions on the part of the clinician are recorded as category eight.

*Category 9:* Client responds correctly and meets the expected level of response pattern.

*Category 10:* Client responds incorrectly; although he apparently tries to meet the demands of the clinician, he does not do so.

Categories nine and ten must be judged in terms of what the clinician asked the client to do, and whether or not his response was appropriate in terms of the clinician's direction, request, command, auditory or visual stimulus. For example, if the clinician asked the client to produce a satisfactory /r/ and his response is /w/, it was incorrect. But if the clinician said: "Make this sound the best you can" (shows letter r), and the client says /w/; he is giving a correct response to the instructions. If the clinician asked the child to repeat a given word correctly three times and he inadvertently repeated it correctly four times, his response was correct, but if he could only repeat it once without an additional auditory model, his response was not correct. If the response satisfied the clinician's criteria for success as identified in the goals, it should be recorded as category nine; if it did not meet this criteria then it should be identified as a ten even though the client was actively attempting to perform the task requested by the clinician. Categories nine and ten are determined by the antecedent behavior of the clinician as well as by the observed behavior of the client.

*Category 11:* Client relates useless information and/or asks irrelevant questions.

This is the type of behavior which is obviously an attempt on the part of the client to avoid following the clinician's instructions because he cannot follow them, because he does not wish to do so, or because he is engaged in "testing" behavior. The most commonly observed types are the client's direct response to the clinician's request with verbal behavior he knows is inappropriate; his attempt to begin a conversation about something irrelevant; or his request for some personal desire to be satisfied as a drink of water, the window open, a different chair, etc. Some common examples are the client's "What time is it?" "When will this lesson be over?" "What are you going to do tonight after you get through working here?" "If I don't do that, will you tell my mother?" "What do you think I saw Big Bird doing on Sesame Street today?" Boone describes a category such as this as a "wastebasket" for the client behavior which is not directly concerned with the goals of the session. The observer should be cautioned against making a value judgement regarding the appropriateness of the occasional social conversation between clinician and client, and record as category eleven all client behaviors that are not related to the tasks identified by the clinician.

*Category 12:* Silence - absence of verbal and relevant motor behavior on the part of both the clinician and the client.

Frequent periods of silence may be observed during the therapy session, and these periods may occur for a variety of reasons. Sometimes there is a need for a brief respite when both clinician and client simply relax in a moment of quiet. On other occasions the silence is a punishing behavior, or it may reflect an unwillingness on the part of the client to follow the clinician's requests. If the client is severely handicapped, the silence may reflect the time necessary for him to make either a verbal or a motor response. On the other hand, the silence may be a "wait" period the clinician has introduced into the therapy before the response is to be attempted, or it may simply represent a skilled clinician's recognition that the client needs a brief period of time before any demand is made of him. The category twelve may be as important as is the pause in conversation or public speaking, or it may be totally irrelevant. In either instance, silence is easy to identify and is recorded as number twelve.

### The ABC System: Recording Procedures

Raw data is collected by observing the therapy session and recording a number on the "Raw Data Collection Sheet" every three seconds, (Figure 1). This number corresponds with the clinician-client interaction occurring at the time of the observation. Therefore, every three seconds a number is placed on the raw data collection sheet.

FIGURE 1

RAW DATA COLLECTION SHEET

Clinician: _____    Disorder: _____

Client: _____    Date: _____

Comments:

_____

_____

_____

_____

_____

The following four basic steps are suggested when learning to use the ABC system.

1. *Learn the categories:* It is necessary to learn the categories so the recorder can identify a behavior by number. A cue work list may help the recorder recall the behaviors quickly. Make a cue card using the following suggested list:

| BEHAVIORAL CATEGORIES |
|---|
| 1. Modifies |
| 2. Instructs |
| 3. Stimulus |
| 4. P/R Positive Reinforcer |
| 5. Punishment |
| 6. R/Inc. - Reinforcement Incorrect |
| 7. Clinician Irrelevant |
| 8. Authority |
| 9. C/R - Correct Response |
| 10. I/R - Incorrect Response |
| 11. Irrelevant Response |
| 12. Silence |

It will help to remember that categories 1-8 are clinician behavior; categories 9-11 are client behavior; and 12 is a joint category, silence.

2. *Learn the time unit:* Categories are identified and recorded at three second intervals. Form the habit of observing and writing the number which identifies the dominant behavior which occurred during the three second interval.

3. *Record the behavior:* The observed behavior is recorded by writing the numbers in the squares shown on the raw data collection sheet. A completed form showing five minutes of interaction is shown in Figure 2.

4. *Analyze the data:* The totals from the raw data collection sheet are then easily and quickly transferred to the ABC Quick Analysis Form, Figure 3. Figure 4 shows the compiled data obtained from Figure 3. From the Quick Analysis Form, the information is then transferred and plotted on the ABC Analysis Form, Figure 5, for setting short and long term objectives. A completed form using the data from Figure 5 is shown in Figure 6.

**FIGURE 2**

COMPLETED

RAW DATA COLLECTION SHEET

Clinician: _____ Disorder: _____

Client: _____ Date: _____

| 3 | 1 | 3 | 9 | 3 | 9 | 12 | 3 | 12 | 12 | 12 | 12 | 12 | 12 | 12 | 7 | 12 | 7 | 11 | 7 |
|---|---|---|---|---|---|----|---|----|----|----|----|----|----|----|---|----|---|----|---|
| 12 | 2 | 3 | 2 | 2 | 7 | 3 | 10 | 2 | 3 | 10 | 3 | 9 | 3 | 9 | 7 | 12 | 3 | 9 | 3 |
| 2 | 2 | 3 | 12 | 3 | 2 | 8 | 3 | 8 | 2 | 3 | 9 | 3 | 12 | 3 | 12 | 3 | 10 | 3 | 12 |
| 7 | 7 | 11 | 7 | 11 | 11 | 11 | 11 | 2 | 3 | 9 | 8 | 8 | 4 | 4 | 3 | 9 | 4 | 3 | 9 |
| 12 | 12 | 12 | 2 | 12 | 12 | 11 | 2 | 8 | 8 | 8 | 8 | 3 | 9 | 8 | 3 | 9 | 3 | 10 | 8 |

Comments:

Child has a light cold and "runny" nose.   Appears to be tired.
_____

_____

_____

_____

_____

**FIGURE 3**

QUICK ANALYSIS FORM

Clinician _____    Date _____

Client _____    Time _____

| Category | Number of Occurrences | Percent of Total |
|----------|----------------------|------------------|
| 1.  (Modifies) | _____ | Total 1s / 100 _____ |
| 2.  (Instructs) | _____ | Total 2s / 100 _____ |
| 3.  (Stimulus) | _____ | Total 3s / 100 _____ |
| 4.  (P/R) | _____ | Total 4s / 100 _____ |
| 5.  (Punishment) | _____ | Total 5s / 100 _____ |
| 6.  (R/Inc.) | _____ | Total 6s / 100 _____ |
| 7.  (Irrelevant) | _____ | Total 7s / 100 _____ |
| 8.  (Authority) | _____ | Total 8s / 100 _____ |
| Subtotal - all clinician behaviors | | _____ |
| 9.  (Correct Response) | _____ | Total 9s / 100 _____ |
| 10. (Inc. Response) | _____ | Total 10s / 100 _____ |
| 11. (Irrel. Response) | _____ | Total 11s / 100 _____ |
| Subtotal - all client behaviors | | _____ |
| 12. (Silence) | _____ | Total 12s / 100 _____ |
| % of sample spent in clinician behavior | | Subtotal A / 100 _____ |
| % of sample spent in client behavior | | Subtotal B / 100 _____ |

Note:  The number of occurrences and percent of total column will be
       identical if a five-minute sample is used--five minutes of
       recorded behavior is equal to 100 recorded observations.

**FIGURE 4**

QUICK ANALYSIS FORM
WITH FIVE MINUTES OF DATA

Clinician _____     Date _____

Client _____    Time _____

| Category | Number of Occurrences | Percent of Total | |
|---|---|---|---|
| 1.  (Modifies) | 1 | Total 1s / 100 | 1 |
| 2.  (Instructs) | 9 | Total 2s / 100 | 9 |
| 3.  (Stimulus) | 25 | Total 3s / 100 | 25 |
| 4.  (P/R) | 3 | Total 4s / 100 | 3 |
| 5.  (Punishment) | 0 | Total 5s / 100 | 0 |
| 6.  (R/Inc.) | 2 | Total 6s / 100 | 2 |
| 7.  (Irrelevant) | 8 | Total 7s / 100 | 8 |
| 8.  (Authority) | 10 | Total 8s / 100 | 10 |
| Subtotal - all clinician behaviors | | 58  65 | |
| 9.  (Correct Response) | 11 | Total 9s / 100 | 11 |
| 10. (Inc. Response) | 4 | Total 10s / 100 | 4 |
| 11. (Irrel. Response) | 7 | Total 11s / 100 | 7 |
| Subtotal - all client behaviors | | 22  18 | |
| 12. (Silence) | 20 | Total 12s / 100 | 20 |
| % of sample spent in clinician behavior | | Subtotal A / 100 | 58 |
| % of sample spent in client behavior | | Subtotal B / 100 | 22 |

Note:  The number of occurrences and percent of total column will be
       identical if a five-minute sample is used--five minutes of
       recorded behavior is equal to 100 recorded observations.

**FIGURE 5**

ABC ANALYSIS FORM

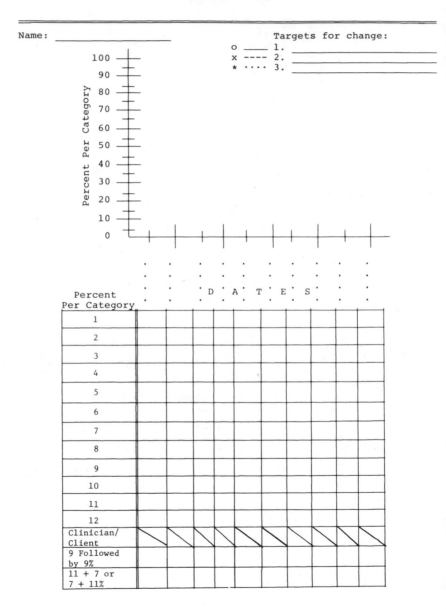

## FIGURE 6

### ABC ANALYSIS FORM

### WITH FIVE MINUTES OF DATA

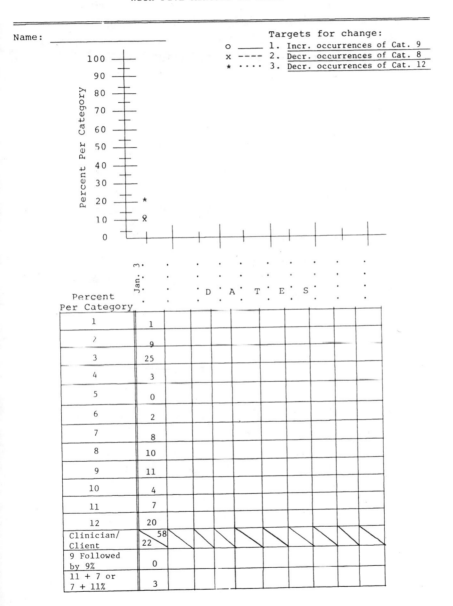

Name: _____

Targets for change:

o ——— 1. Incr. occurrences of Cat. 9
x – – – – 2. Decr. occurrences of Cat. 8
* · · · · 3. Decr. occurrences of Cat. 12

| Percent Per Category | Jan. 3 | D A T E S | | | | | | |
|---|---|---|---|---|---|---|---|---|
| 1 | 1 | | | | | | | |
| 2 | 9 | | | | | | | |
| 3 | 25 | | | | | | | |
| 4 | 3 | | | | | | | |
| 5 | 0 | | | | | | | |
| 6 | 2 | | | | | | | |
| 7 | 8 | | | | | | | |
| 8 | 10 | | | | | | | |
| 9 | 11 | | | | | | | |
| 10 | 4 | | | | | | | |
| 11 | 7 | | | | | | | |
| 12 | 20 | | | | | | | |
| Clinician/ Client | 58 / 22 | | | | | | | |
| 9 Followed by 9% | 0 | | | | | | | |
| 11 + 7 or 7 + 11% | 3 | | | | | | | |

From the analysis the following conclusion can be drawn: the clinician shows a poor stimulus-response time ratio. During the five minute segment of therapy the clinician stimulated the client for 75 seconds (25 x 3) for a client return of 45 seconds of response time (15 x 3). Second, the use of categories 7 and 11, Irrelevant Talk by both clinician and client, is high. It equals 15 observations which is equivalent to the response time of the client. When time spent in Silence is examined, it is found that 20 observations were recorded, equalizing 60 seconds (20 x 3) or exactly one-fifth of the therapy time sample.

Also, it should be noted that the clinician uses a great deal of authority to control the child, ten occurrences within the five-minute segment.

Increases and decreases in all behavioral categories are recorded on the bottom half of the ABC Analysis Form; therefore, all behaviors can be analyzed and/or plotted at any time. However, it is recommended that the clinician and supervisor set specific goals relating to three categories, plot them on the graph (usually weekly) and determine at a later time if the established objectives are being achieved. It is obvious that an increase in the usage of one category means a decrease in some other category or categories and vice versa.

Specific goals which could be agreed on from this sample of therapy and plotted for long term analysis are:

1. Increase the number of occurrences of Category 9, Correct Client Response.

2. Decrease the number of occurrences of Category 8, Use of Authority.

3. Decrease the number of occurrences of Category 12, Silence.

Using the three previously stated targets (objectives) for change, Figure 7 shows an example of ten five-minute samples of

**FIGURE 7**

ABC ANALYSIS FORM

WITH TEN FIVE-MINUTE THERAPY SEGMENTS

Name: _____

Targets for change:
- o _____ 1. Incr. occurrences of Cat. 9
- x - - - - 2. Decr. occurrences of Cat. 8
- ★ · · · · 3. Decr. occurrences of Cat. 12

| Percent Per Category | Jan. 3 | Jan. 10 | Jan. 17 | Jan. 24 | Feb. 7 | Feb. 14 | Feb. 21 | Feb. 28 | Mar. 7 | Mar. 14 |
|---|---|---|---|---|---|---|---|---|---|---|
| 1 | 1 | 0 | 2 | 3 | 2 | 0 | 4 | 0 | 1 | 0 |
| 2 | 9 | 8 | 10 | 10 | 11 | 14 | 10 | 8 | 9 | 5 |
| 3 | 25 | 25 | 23 | 20 | 19 | 16 | 15 | 19 | 17 | 19 |
| 4 | 3 | 7 | 6 | 8 | 10 | 11 | 9 | 12 | 11 | 9 |
| 5 | 0 | 3 | 1 | 2 | 0 | 0 | 4 | 0 | 1 | 0 |
| 6 | 2 | 2 | 2 | 3 | 2 | 1 | 2 | 1 | 0 | 0 |
| 7 | 8 | 6 | 9 | 7 | 4 | 3 | 5 | 1 | 2 | 2 |
| 8 | 10 | 7 | 12 | 10 | 2 | 5 | 3 | 0 | 3 | 3 |
| 9 | 11 | 11 | 15 | 9 | 21 | 18 | 20 | 35 | 35 | 40 |
| 10 | 4 | 3 | 3 | 4 | 5 | 3 | 4 | 1 | 0 | 3 |
| 11 | 7 | 3 | 0 | 5 | 8 | 5 | 3 | 3 | 1 | 0 |
| 12 | 20 | 25 | 17 | 19 | 16 | 24 | 21 | 20 | 20 | 20 |
| Clinician/Client | 58 / 22 | 58 / 17 | 65 / 18 | 63 / 18 | 50 / 34 | 50 / 26 | 52 / 27 | 41 / 39 | 44 / 36 | 38 / 42 |
| 9 Followed by 9% | 0 | 2 | 6 | 4 | 8 | 6 | 8 | 9 | 10 | 12 |
| 11 + 7 or 7 + 11% | 3 | 4 | 0 | 2 | 4 | 3 | 1 | 1 | 1 | 0 |

therapy sessions. From this data it can be seen that two of the three objectives are being met. First, there is a steady increase in the use of Category 9, Client Responds Correctly. The second objective which is being met is a decrease in the use of Category 8, Using Authority. The objective which is not being met is a decrease in Silence, Category 12.

### The ABC System: Summary

Student clinician and supervisor spend a great deal of time attempting to change clinical behavior. In this era of accountability it is necessary to determine objectively what is occurring, and later determine if progress has been achieved. The ABC System allows clinicians and supervisors to quantify and examine clinical interaction. They are able to plan jointly for increases and decreases in specific behavior and determine if the planned objectives are being met. The ABC System provides a useful tool for identifying clinical behaviors and revealing clinical behavioral changes which occur as students progress in their clinical experience.

### Time Required for Supervisory Observation

Studies have been completed relating to the length of time required to obtain a representative sample of student clinician-client interaction. Boone and Goldberg (1969) reveal that a random five-minute segment of the middle twenty minutes of a half-hour therapy session offered as much information as scoring the total twenty-minute session.

Boone and Prescott (1972b), using the Boone and Prescott 10 Category System, concluded that when a therapy session was studied, the first five minutes and the last five minutes of a half-hour therapy session were not representative of the whole session. These segments contained less stimulus-response-reward data and more rapport related responses than did the rest of the session.

Schubert and Laird (1975) investigated the length of time required to obtain a representative sample of student clinician and client interaction when using the ABC System. The results of the study show that when five different three-minute segments of therapy were studied no significant differences occurred in behavior. The fifteen minutes studied excluded the initial and final five minutes of therapy session. This information supports the position that behaviors occurring in the therapy session are very stable and reoccur at a very rapid rate. This means that experimenters, supervisors, and clinicians can use data from three minutes of therapy for evaluation and be confident that they have a representative sample of student clinician and client interaction.

### Comparison of the ABC and Boone-Prescott 10 Category System

A study by Schubert and Glick (1975) revealed that the two most commonly used observation systems in speech pathology were the ABC System and Boone-Prescott 10-Category System. Preceding this time, an investigation was completed which compared these two systems.

Although the Boone and Prescott System differs from the ABC System in total number of behavioral categories, certain categories within the two systems are similar. Eight categories within the two systems are similar. The similar categories are as follows:

| Boone and Prescott System | ABC System |
|---|---|
| 1. Explain and Describe | 2. Instruction and Demonstration |
| 2. Model and Instruction | 3. Auditory and/or Visual Stimulation |
| 3. Good Evaluative | 4. Auditory and/or Visual Positive Reinforcement of Client's Correct Sound |
| 4. Bad Evaluative | 5. Auditory and/or Visual Punishment of Client's Incorrect Sound |
| 5. Neutral-Social | 7. Clinician Relating Irrelevant Information |
| 6. Correct Response | 9. Client Responds Correctly |
| 7. Incorrect Response | 10. Client Responds Incorrectly |
| 8. Inappropriate-Social | 11. Client Relating Irrelevant Information |

The major difference between the two systems is the criteria for recording behaviors. When the Boone and Prescott System is used, recording of data is determined by change in behavior; while recording of data is time-based when the ABC System is used.

The results of the study revealed that there was no significant difference when the total number of observations from the two systems was compared. Basically, the two systems yielded the same number of behaviors. When the rank order of the eight similar categories of the two systems was compared, a perfect positive correlation was attained, as the ranking of both systems was identical.

Both the Boone and Prescott System and the ABC System will provide the student clinician and supervisor with much information about the therapy session. Both systems are useful in changing and improving student clinician behavior by providing objective information pertaining to clinician-client interaction.

## Summary

An historical review of the techniques used to identify and record specific behaviors was presented in this chapter. The development of the Flanders' Interaction Analysis System and its influence on other systems, such as the Analysis of Behavior of Clinicians (ABC) System, has been reviewed.

The ABC System, its development, its use, and its procedures are given in detail. Along with specific directions for usage, all forms and forms with complete examples are demonstrated visually. A sample of a therapy session approximately three to five minutes in duration was shown as the length of time required to obtain a representative sample of student clinician-client interaction.

The ABC System and the Boone and Prescott 10 Category System were compared. In essence, these two systems reveal approximately the same data in reference to clinician-client interaction. Both systems are extremely useful in analyzing and modifying student clinician interaction.

## Questions and Issues

1. What is meant by "interaction analysis?" For how long and for what purposes have interaction analysis systems been used?

2. In what ways are the ABC and the Boone-Prescott 10 Category systems similar? In what ways are the two systems different? Determine the liabilities and assets of the two systems.

3. Does research concerning the ABC System and the Boone-Prescott 10 Category System support the concept that the two systems are reliable interaction analysis systems? Explain.

4. Discuss the length of time a supervisor or other individuals collecting information through the use of an interaction analysis system should spend collecting data. What exceptions might there be to a general rule regarding this matter? Justify and explain both the rule and the exceptions.

5. Which categories in the ABC System are the most valuable? Why? Which categories are the least useful? What suggestion do you have for changing and improving the system?

# CHAPTER 4

## EVALUATION OF STUDENT CLINICIANS

### Introduction

This chapter will concern itself with the evaluation of clinical behaviors of student clinicians without the use of objective evaluation systems. Observation systems and their use are presented in Chapter 3.

Evaluations are necessary to determine the progress of the student toward competence in the professional field he has chosen. In speech pathology, the student clinician is evaluated in reference to his ability to establish and accomplish therapeutic goals which are appropriate for his client.

### Grading System

Most educational systems provide for the assignment of some type of a final grade or statement at the end of each grading period for the student clinician concerning his progress in practicum and academic courses. The final statement or the cumulation of grades from the grading period represents an evaluation of the student's skill and progress during a specified length of time. More often than not, this grade is represented by a letter (A, B, C, D, F) and describes the quality of a student's performance in relationship to his peers as determined by evaluation criteria established by the institution and/or the supervisor.

The letter grade achieved by the student clinician in a practicum course is an assessment of clinical performance which has been assigned by the clinical supervisor. The supervisor makes a final evaluation and decision represented basically by the student's therapy techniques and procedures. Many separate criteria usually are included in what is meant by therapy techniques and procedures. These criteria will be explored in detail later within this chapter.

Students, supervisors, professors, employers, and many other people make judgments and decisions by using the grade assigned to students in both practicum and academic courses. Often the grades assigned to students in practicum courses receive more attention than grades assigned to students in academic courses. Obviously, this is true of prospective employers seeking competent clinicians. Letter grades assigned to students are also used for admission into graduate programs, eligibility for financial awards, peer and self-evaluation, and a variety of other things. The clinical supervisor must be aware of the multi-use of comparative letter grading.

It is important that the definition of each letter grade be specifically stated and that the stated definition be used when making letter grade assignments. The following definitions are suggested for use when assigning letter grades to students in practicum courses in speech pathology.

A—Marked excellence, superior achievement

B—Above average

C—Average

D—Below average, but passing

F—Failure

It is important that these definitions be used. Too often students who are doing average work (C) are assigned a letter grade of B, thereby distorting the definition. This procedure is not fair to the student nor to people who are attempting to evaluate prospective clinicians for future employment. The supervisor who awards a letter grade of B to a student who has performed according to what is defined as average, or C behavior, is deceiving both the student and those who attempt to evaluate the student's clinical achievements.

Although the potential advantages of comparative grading just discussed should be kept in mind, the possible disadvantages should be considered. Educators opposed to comparative grading provide the following criticisms of this method.

1.  Emphasis on grades limits creativity and individuality of expression. Grades may discourage rather than encourage learning that is personally relevant to the student.

2.  Grades place too much pressure on the student. Learning should be an enjoyable experience; grades are too often tension-creating experiences. Students should not be forced to compete with each other to earn high grades.

3.  When working for high grades is stressed, much of what has been learned will be forgotten as soon as the grade is achieved.

4.  Instructors are too authoritative. Students are forced to "spit back" exactly what the book or instructor said with the fear of a low grade being assigned.

Since the onset of more liberal educational procedures, the letter grade has again come under criticism. Some departments allow students to choose their course of study without many curricular requirements. Students are often under a contract system to supply a specific amount of work for a specific grade. This emphasizes quantity and minimizes evaluations of quality. A contract approach lessens public comparison and competition among students.

Many institutions and departments have increased the number of pass-fail or satisfactory-unsatisfactory hours allowed to be used toward graduation requirement. The appeal of pass-fail grading is based on the fact that it reduces pressure and is thought likely to encourage study because the student wants to learn, not just obtain a high grade.

When this point is made, it implies that learning for personal value and learning to obtain a good grade are mutually exclusive. According to Gardner (1961), the best way to motivate people to make the most of their abilities is to establish and enforce standards. The standard in pass-fail systems draws toward the level of those who just pass. Markle (1964) states that pass-fail tends to decrease student effort because of the lowest-common-denominator effect. To assure the majority of the students passing, instructors revise their programs for the slowest students in the group. This eventually leads to programs that most students can complete fairly easily, but becomes over-simplified and repetitious.

Another disadvantage of the pass-fail system is unreliability. Whenever a few categories are used such as the two in a pass-fail system, the results are less consistent. The likelihood that a given instructor will assign a different grade on a second evaluation of borderline students, or that different instructors will assign different grades, increases as the number of categories decreases.

If fair and objective criteria are applied to a measuring device, the result is likely to be a valid and reliable sample of academic behavior. In clinical practicums, the letter grade represents the demonstration by a student of the ability to engage in a sustained and meaningful interaction with a client.

Included in this evaluation are likely to be such criteria as:

— Effectiveness of therapy

— Knowledge of dismissal criteria

— Knowledge of diagnostic procedures

— Ability to establish and maintain rapport

— Ability to relate and communicate with client and other people

— Ability to establish appropriate therapy goals

— Ability to evaluate progress of the client

A grade is assigned to the student indicating his progress during a specified length of time. Ideally, the expectations and criticisms have been explained by the supervisor and have been understood by the student clinician. The final grade should reflect the success and failure the student has had in attempting to meet the established requirements of the course. The advantages of using letter grades are summarized as follows:

— Letter grades provide feedback which often functions as reinforcement. This is an essential part of learning.

— Letter grades help to guarantee that a student will master basic facts and skills and this will lead to a mastery of concepts and general abilities.

— Letter grades motivate the student to learn in a more detailed manner. This helps to assure those concerned individuals that the material will be remembered.

— Letter grades supply specific feedback which permits the student to compete against himself.

— Letter grades require that the supervisor be specific in identifying liabilities and assets of the student. This assists the supervisor in improving his own performance.

Letter grading forces upon the evaluator a more systematic method of evaluating students. Many departments which have tried to use the satisfactory-unsatisfactory system of grading have returned to the previous method of grading, that of letter grades. The main reason for this is that minimal difficulty was found in identifying the student who was doing unsatisfactory work, but no way exists to reflect the difference between the marginally adequate student clinician and the superior competent person. With the satisfactory-unsatisfactory method of grading there is no way to indicate growth and energy versus minimal advancement and the "just-get-by" student. The satisfactory-unsatisfactory grade in professional courses encourages minimal effort and becomes discouraging to the good student.

Even though many students and faculty members advocate eliminating the ABC grading system in favor of satisfactory-unsatisfactory grading, this is not likely to happen. The need for a descriptive and qualitative measure of student progress is necessary.

## Brief Early History of Evaluative Criteria

Criteria used in evaluating the proficiency of clinicians have been widely discussed by members of the profession. The early articles included broad concepts and recommendations for an accepted procedure, and included personal characteristics not directly related to practicum.

Powers (1956) listed numerous evaluative criteria with which the supervisor could evaluate the student clinician. The evaluative criteria included six main divisions:

1. Organization of speech correction programs

2. Examination and diagnosis of cases

3. Speech therapy

4. Professional relationships

5. Personal characteristics

6. Professional attitude and ethics

The six main divisions were supplemented with numerous other criteria. The supervisor was to mark the evaluative criteria either satisfactory or unsatisfactory.

In 1958, Herbert published a list of evaluative criteria. In comparison to Powers' criteria, Herbert used only three major areas:

1. Personal qualities

2. Professional qualities

3. Teaching performance

Within the three major areas, Herbert used less than one hundred evaluative criteria compared to approximately twice that number used by Powers.

In 1964, the American Speech and Hearing Association with Villarreal as the seminar editor, published guidelines for supervision of clinical practicum. The forty-four page publication dealing exclusively with supervision, discusses various aspects of the supervisory process. The authors stated:

Until objective guidelines become available, however, reliance must be placed on professional judgment of the experienced clinical supervisor. Within this context, the following criteria are suggested as incidence of clinical performance by which the supervisor may assess the student clinician's clinical performance.

1. The ability to establish rapport with patients

2. The ability to demonstrate sufficient knowledge of diagnostic and therapeutic techniques appropriate to the patient's problem

3. The ability to modify and adapt examination and treatment procedures in appropriate ways to meet the needs of specific clinical situations

4. The ability to recognize problems of the individual as a whole and make appropriate referrals when necessary

5. The ability to demonstrate a working concept of the total therapeutic process with respect to speech, hearing, and language problems

6. The ability to apply therapeutic techniques to effectuate desired changes in the patient's behavior which often involves motivating the patient to modify his own behavior

Schubert (1967, 1968) conducted a survey to determine the criteria most frequently used in evaluating student clinicians. Responses from thirty-one training institutions throughout the United States indicated a range of four to forty-seven criteria. The mean number of criteria used by these schools was twenty-two. The twenty criteria reported most frequently were translated into behavioral terms and were as follows:

1. Demonstrates an ability to accomplish identified goals

2. Shows an understanding of the client's speech problems and his secondary problems

3. Establishes rapport

4. Exhibits professional attitudes

5. Displays adequate personal appearance and hygiene

6. Plans therapy to accomplish goals of therapy

7. Attends to therapy setting and clinical materials

8. Demonstrates knowledge of communication problems

9. Demonstrates reliability-dependability

10. Uses appropriate voice, speech, and language

11. Keeps adequate records and writes satisfactory reports

12. Accepts criticism and carries out recommendations of the supervisor

13. Exhibits emotional stability

14. Establishes appropriate goals

15. Is skillful in motivating the client

16. Engages in self-evaluation

17. Evaluates progress of the client

18. Works individually

19. Gives proper time to review

20. Provides for carryover

More recent research suggests that the clinical supervisor use criteria to evaluate the clinician which have a direct influence on changing the speech pattern of the client.

### Evaluation Criteria in Clinical Practicum

It is the responsibility of the clinical supervisor to make judgments and decisions about the capabilities and weaknesses of the student clinician. The supervisor must have a means for bringing the clinician's attention to these behaviors. The supervisor must communicate objective and subjective criticism to the student clinician.

The number of evaluative criteria and the procedure for obtaining this information is extremely diverse. Most training institutions have experimented with using many different evaluation forms during the past few years. This continuous changing process is necessary as the profession and society changes. Evaluation criteria change and procedures for collecting the information are modified. Criteria which was extremely important a few years ago when evaluating the student clinician may not be as important today. An example of this is the dress of the clinician. It was very important in most clinical settings that the male clinician wear a tie and suit, the female clinician wear a dress, or skirt and blouse. Today it remains important that student clinicians be dressed clean and neat, but the formal dress is not as important as it was a few years ago, and in a weighted evaluation system this criteria would not be valued as high as it was in the past.

Geoffrey (1973) notes that when the clinical supervisor is able to observe the therapy session frequently, the verbal critique is most often used, but when supervision is less frequent the rating scale and written critiques are used most often.

When evaluative criteria or rating scales are used, it is important that the terms and statements used on these systems be understood. Terms and labels need to be defined, either verbally or in writing, so that both the student clinician and supervisor are able to communicate. Also, it is important that within a particular training institution the terms being used for evaluation purposes have the same meaning from one supervisor to another. Without this unanimity a student needs to interpret what one supervisor means as opposed to what another supervisor means. A clear understanding facilitates clear communication among supervisors.

The purpose of a list of competencies, or evaluative criteria, is to provide feedback to the student clinician in an effort to help him modify his behavior in such a way that he will become a more effective clinician. The criteria employed in this evaluation list must include the important and relevant items. It is possible to develop a list of competency-based skills which would number one or two hundred items. However, such a lengthy listing is very time consuming to complete, often the supervisor cannot collect enough information in the time allotted for observation to complete the form. Also, many of the items to be evaluated would be of minor concern. It is much more valuable to decide on 15-30 items which are to be used to evaluate the clinician and proceed with the development of a precise and clear criterion listing. The criteria used must be meaningful to the clinician. The student clinician needs to be able to identify and understand his clinical weaknesses and strengths through the use of the evaluation criteria and the explanation of this criteria as discussed with him by his supervisor.

Before creating a list of criteria from which the student clinician can be evaluated, the following questions must be answered:

1. Does the evaluative criteria used represent the important clinical skills needed by the speech clinicians?

2. Does the list include an adequate number of items to evaluate the clinician and session? An ample number of items must be included to insure a fair assessment.

3. Is the list of items used to evaluate the student clinician too lengthy and/or include irrelevant criteria?

4. Can some of the items listed be evaluated in an objective manner?

5. Is the terminology defined or will it be orally explained? The terminology used in defining the criteria should not interfere with the performance or evaluation of the clinician.

6. Do the evaluative items focus on clinical skills?

7. Will the complete evaluation form provide useful feedback to the clinician?

Answers to the above seven questions should be yes, except for question three. With consideration of these questions in mind, one can develop a form to be used by the supervisor and student for the purpose of improving clinical skills. These forms are usually referred to as a rating form, rating scale, evaluation scale, evaluation form, evaluation criteria, clinical skills checklist, and clinical competency checklist.

Typical evaluation criteria used to assess clinical competencies of student clinicians are as follows:

1. Use of clinical and diagnostic information

2. Acceptance and use of the clinical supervisor's recommendations

3. Development of appropriate lesson plans

4. Evaluation of lesson plans following a therapy session.

5. Use of original and appropriate therapy techniques

6. Skill in using mechanical equipment; skill in using clinical and diagnostic materials

7. Skill in establishing rapport with clients

8. Ability to write clinical reports (letters, evaluations, notes, etc.)

9. Ability to establish and re-establish appropriate goals and objectives for clients

10. Ability to motivate the client

11. Ability to control the therapy session

12. Cooperation with other service agencies

13. Use of approptiate verbal communication

14. Asks meaningful questions in an effort to obtain useful information

15. Use of learning principles

16. Dependability

17. Skill in listening and observing

18. Skill in using discipline

19. Makes effective use of time

20. Uses knowledge of theory and research in the clinical setting

The above twenty evaluation criteria are not all inclusive. In fact, a detailed list of evaluation criteria could be more than one hundred items. However, such a lengthy list of criteria is usually very difficult and time consuming to use. Other criteria which have been used when evaluating student clinicians, but which focus less directly on clinical skills are clinician cleans up the therapy room following the therapy session, dress and grooming of clinician, and clinician cooperates with classmates. It is not that the previous criteria may not have an overall effect on the client's behavior, but this criteria and similar criteria may not affect the client in a direct manner. However, it is important to note, for example, that the dress and grooming of a clinician may have a very direct effect on the success the clinician will have or is having with a particular client. When this is the situation, the importance of these criteria and similar criteria must be recognized by the student clinician and supervisor.

**FIGURE 8**

University of North Dakota
Speech and Hearing Clinic

EVALUATION OF CLINICAL PRACTICUM

Student Clinician _____  Client _____

Supervisor _____  Date _____

Key

| Letter Grade | Terminology | Point Value |
|---|---|---|
| A | Exceptional, Excellent, Superior | 5 |
| B | Very good, Above average | 4 |
| C | Satisfactory, Acceptable, Average | 3 |
| D | Marginal, Weak, Below average | 2 |
| F | Poor, Failing, Not acceptable | 1 |

| | 5 | 4 | 3 | 2 | 1 |
|---|---|---|---|---|---|
| 1. Use of clinical and diagnostic information . . . . . . . . . . . . . . | | | | | |
| 2. Use of supervisor's suggestions and recommendations . . . . . . . . . . . | | | | | |
| 3. Development of appropriate lesson plans . . . . . . . . . . . . . . . . | | | | | |
| 4. Self-evaluation of therapy sessions . . . | | | | | |
| 5. Use of therapy techniques . . . . . . . . | | | | | |
| 6. Skill in using mechanical equipment . . . | | | | | |
| 7. Skill in establishing rapport . . . . . . | | | | | |
| 8. Written communication skills . . . . . . | | | | | |

| | 5 | 4 | 3 | 2 | 1 |
|---|---|---|---|---|---|
| 9. Ability to establish appropriate therapeutic goals and objectives . . . . . . . . . . . . . . . | | | | | |
| 10. Ability to motivate client . . . . . . . . | | | | | |
| 11. Skill in controling therapy session. . . . | | | | | |
| 12. Cooperation with service agencies. . . . . | | | | | |
| 13. Use of appropriate verbal communication. . . . . . . . . . . . . . | | | | | |
| 14. Asks meaningful questions, seeks useful information. . . . . . . . . . . . . . . | | | | | |
| 15. Uses learning principles . . . . . . . . . | | | | | |
| 16. Dependability. . . . . . . . . . . . . . . | | | | | |
| 17. Skill in listening and observing . . . . . | | | | | |
| 18. Skill in using discipline. . . . . . . . . | | | | | |
| 19. Uses time effectively. . . . . . . . . . . | | | | | |
| 20. Uses knowledge of theory and research. . . | | | | | |
| 21. Is able to work independently with minimal supervision. . . . . . . . . . . | | | | | |
| 22. Demonstrates emotional stability . . . . . | | | | | |
| 23. Uses appropriate feedback. . . . . . . . . | | | | | |
| 24. Recognizes unique characteristics of the client . . . . . . . . . . . . . . . | | | | | |
| 25. Modifies therapy according to needs of the client. . . . . . . . . . . . . . | | | | | |

Recommendations:

_____

_____

_____

_____

An example of an evaluation scale is presented in Figure 8. With this example, a point value is used. Many supervisors will prefer a similar form, but rather than assigning a point value they will use a check-off system. Here the supervisor would check an appropriate box labeled above average, average, or below average for each evaluative criteria. Either system works and in reality the information is translated by the clinician and supervisor into the same final product. The Final evaluation includes a method of comparing one student with other student clinicians, an individual evaluation of a particular student, a guide for communication, and a tool for determining a grade.

When using evaluation forms, it is necessary to evaluate the competencies of the student according to the expected performance of a student for that particular level. Therefore, a third alternative for evaluation is possible. In addition to using numbers (1, 2, 3, 4, 5) or using average, above average, or below average, the supervisor may use the following terms: expected performance for a student at this level, (EP), unusually good performance for student at this level (UGP), and poorer than average performance for a student at this level (PAP). Here again a check is placed in the appropriate box following the criteria listing.

The purpose of student evaluations include: it helps the student to recognize his professional assets and liabilities; it serves as a means of changing and improving clinical skills of the student; it supplies a means of demonstrating accountability for both the student clinician and supervisor; it provides a record of the student's clinical skills and progress for future reference; it serves as an aid when counseling students; and it is a means of helping the student to self-evaluate. Much of the worth of any evaluation depends upon the relationship existing between the student and the clinical supervisor.

Students need to be evaluated periodically because such evaluations reflect areas of performance which need to be modified and improved. Continuous evaluation, both internal and external, needs to be part of the clinical training program for all students. It is only through continuous evaluation and reception of feedback that the student can obtain maximum benefit from his clinical experience.

The questions which no evaluation form can answer are those that ask "why". For example, "Why is the student clinician doing a poor job in using available information regarding a client who is assigned to him?" Perhaps the answer is a lack of concern for the client or in a broader sense, a lack of concern and interest in the profession. Other possible answers include insufficient knowledge about how to use the information and inadequate training concerning the use of this information. The important point here is that the evaluation form can help the supervisor and clinician to identify the incompetency if this area is deficient, and once identified, a plan to change the situation can be implemented.

When evaluation forms are employed, they should be used in conjunction with oral and written feedback. Using this procedure, evaluation forms can be used several times during a particular practicum experience. Evaluation forms should be designed with this procedure in mind. Also, when evaluation forms are to be used by a supervisor, they should be explained to the student and used early during the practicum experience. In this way the student understands the specific purpose of the evaluation form and how it is to be used in helping him become a competent clinician. Regular use of the form allows the student and supervisor to focus and refocus on behaviors which need to be modified over time.

## Summary

Assigning grades to students is the responsibility of the clinical supervisor. Also, it is the responsibility and professional obligation of the supervisor to assign the grade achieved by a student to that student. If a student is functioning at an average level he should then be assigned the letter grade which defines average, in most situations that letter grade is a C. A supervisor who does not do this is cheating the student, prospective employers, and the profession.

When evaluating student clinicians and determining grades for students, it is important that criteria meaningful to the clinical task be used. If criteria are used which do not measure clinical competencies, the result will be a false evaluation. It appears that letter grading is a more descriptive and better form of evaluating clinical skills than is a bifunctional system, such as pass-fail.

Evaluation forms are used at many institutions as one method of providing feedback to student clinicians. A single evaluation form does not exist that meets the needs of all institutions. Supervisors may want to develop their own forms. Evaluation forms may be developed for specific types of disorders. The important thing to remember when developing and using any evaluation form is that the form focuses on clinical skills and that the form aids the clinician and supervisor in improving the clinical skills of the clinician.

## Questions and Issues

1. It is the responsibility and obligation of the clinical supervisor to assign the appropriate letter grade earned by the student to the student. A student who has earned a grade of D should not be assigned a letter grade of C-. Discuss the ramifications of these statements.

2. It is possible that some evaluation criteria may be more important and more meaningful with one client (Client A) than it is with another client (Client B). Explain.

3. When pass-fail grading has been used in clinical competency based courses, it has often met with unsatisfactory results. Discuss why this is true and how the situation may be improved.

4. Discuss the statement, "I know what I said, but did you understand what I said?" Consider the meaning of the word "acceptable" in your discussion of the aforementioned statement.

5. Discuss the values of using an evaluation form when supervising student clinicians. When evaluation forms are used, how often should they be completed by the supervisor?

# CHAPTER 5

## REPORT WRITING

### Importance and Purpose

The importance of report writing cannot be over-emphasized. The written report serves to communicate ideas, thoughts, progress, and recommendations. These issues are critical to the supervisor, the clinician, the client, and other professionals.

Many reports become part of the personal field of the client. The report may serve as a record for future referrals; it may serve as a legal document; or information may be extracted from the report and used for research purposes.

The writing of the report is important in a personal way. That is, the report represents the writer's personal communicative skills, his use and knowledge of the English language, and his patience in report writing. Often, professionals judge other professionals as competent or incompetent based on communication in report writing. The following outline includes the necessary concepts which need to be considered when organizing and writing most reports.

I.  The purpose of the report is to communicate:

A. Ideas

B. Thoughts

C. Observations

D. Impressions

E. Results

F. Recommendations

II. The major uses of the report are for:

    A. Planning

    B. Record for future referral

    C. Legal purposes

    D. Research purposes

III. The report is usually directed toward:

    A. Other professional workers

    B. Parents

    C. School personnel

    D. Others

Although each clinic usually has a format which is preferred for the writing of reports, common areas exist which should be included in report writing. Of course, areas need to be included, excluded, or modified depending on the type and function of the report. For example, a diagnostic report is not written in exactly the same way as a progress report. Following is a list of headings which should be considered for inclusion when accumulating information and writing a report:

## IDENTIFYING INFORMATION

— Patient's name

— Patient's birthdate

— Patient's birthplace

— Patient's age

— Patient's address

— Patient's telephone number

- Parental information

    Age of parents

    Employment of parents

- Date of evaluation
- Clinic number
- Referral source
- Reason for referral

## INVESTIGATIVE INFORMATION

- Background information
- Oral examination
- Hearing examination
- Speech evaluation

    Articulation

    Rate

    Fluency (disfluency)

- Language evaluation
- Voice evaluation
- Clinical Impressions
- Recommendations

### Writing the Report

The experience of report writing and rewriting, to most of us, does not represent enjoyable memories. In fact, to most people these memories could be compared to nightmares. The painful experience of having a report returned by a supervisor with the report almost completely rewritten is not uncommon.

The above situation is true because formal training in report writing is lacking. Typically, the student learns to write reports through an elaborate trial and error method. Usually, to make things worse, the trial and error method does not teach the clinician to become an effective report writer. First, the clinician does not write enough reports during clinical training to become an efficient report writer. Ten or twenty reports which have been corrected and recorrected by the clinical supervisor are not sufficient to teach and to develop the necessary skills needed in report writing. Second, the clinical supervisor does not have the time to teach the skill of report writing effectively. The supervisor must establish priorities concerning his time and the clinician's time. The priority is almost always that of teaching clinical skills to the clinician rather than the writing skills.

It would be wise for the supervisor to devote some time, which is normally devoted to clinical demonstrations or observations of therapy, to explanations and discussions of report writing. The supervisor should remind the clinician that correct grammatical organization should be used. Tense, agreement, and construction of verbs are important in the relaying of correct messages. It often creates a problem if the writer and the reader misunderstand the verb. Equally important is the correct use of pronoun and antecedent. Pronouns, like verbs, must agree in number and case. The clinician should exhibit a working knowledge of sentence formation. Sentences which are too long and complex should be avoided. These sentences cause misunderstandings and the tendency to be incorrect is greater.

Words that are used should be recognized as words in the English language. The clinician or writer should not try to create his own words. Jargon, clichés, and ambiguous words should be avoided. Ambiguous words have no meaning to the reader as he tries to interpret the message.

A misconception in report writing is that personal pronouns should never be used. When the natural flow of the report calls for the use of a personal pronoun, it should be used. This does not mean that every sentence should include a personal pronoun, but it does mean that the terms examiners, clinician, tester, therapist, and researcher may be more adequately represented by a personal pronoun. Words like "I", and "you" are part of the English language and do not need to be excluded when writing reports.

The time spent in grammatical review will be well spent and can save much rewriting by both the clinician and the supervisor. Not only will this formal procedure save time, but the learning is likely to be more effective than when the clinician tries to rewrite the report using the supervisor's written comments.

Abbreviations should be used sparingly. The obvious reason for this is that the reader may not be familiar with the abbreviation, or even worse, the reader may misinterpret the abbreviation thereby creating the possibility of further incorrect communication and additional related problems. The saving of space and the writer's time is not a justifiable excuse for using abbreviations which are critical to the written communication process. Abbreviations should not be used in report writing unless the writer is sure that the abbreviation will convey the meaning which was intended.

The length of the written report is dictated by its purpose and the amount of information available about the client. If a communication has been received requesting information regarding the progress of a client, then a report regarding the progress should be written. In this case, information concerning extraneous information should be excluded. One might ask, "Why not include all of the available information?" It is very costly to include five pages of information when only one is needed. Cost may also be incurred by the typist typing the information and the reproduction and storage of the information.

Next, when a colleague receives more information than he requests or needs, he may not sift through the information. If he does, it is costly due to the unnecessary time commitment. Also, this type of reporting may interfere with future requests and future referrals by the annoyed colleague.

Consider for whom the report is being written. A medical doctor, an orthodontist, an elementary school principal, or a parent may request the information. Take into account the person's needs, knowledge of terminology and, if known, his education. Again, these are only a few of the many items which should be considered when writing a report for a particular person or agency.

In most cases, the clinical report should be written in narrative form. Sentences should be clear and to the point. Choose each word carefully, making certain that you have chosen the words to convey what you mean. If you do not know the meaning of a word, technical or nontechnical, look the word up, examine the definitions, and decide if the word means what you want to say.

Often it is necessary to report observations of clients. When this is done, the actual observation should be reported, as opposed to using a term which implies many different behaviors. Rather than saying "John was hyperactive," the writer should say, "John moved from chair to chair throughout the one-half hour session." Following the actual description of what occurred, the writer may then use the term which he believes defines the behavior. Therefore, in this case, the writer would state, "John moved from chair to chair throughout the one-half hour session demonstrating hyperactive behavior."

All reports should be concluded with the names and signatures of the people who completed the report. The names should be typed on the report and the signature should appear just above the typed name. Along with the names should be the degree and title of the person. An example is as follows:

*Glen W. Smith*

Glen W. Smith, Ph.D.
Speech Pathologist
Associate Professor

## Summary

The do's of report writing are presented as a partial summary to this material.

The do's of report writing:

— Devote an appropriate amount of time and effort to writing reports.

— Give a high priority to learning report writing skills.

— When preparing the report, consider the specific purpose for which the report is being prepared.

— Include only the necessary and requested information within the report.

— Consider for whom the report is being written.

— Write the report in narrative form.

— Use words which express the meaning you want to convey.

— Report the observation rather than using a technical term.

— Be specific and avoid vague generalities when reporting observations.

— Write reports which are clear and to the point.

— Eliminate redundancies.

— Check your report for correct grammatical organization including tense agreement; verb construction; pronoun and antecedent; agreement in number; split infinitives; participial phrases; complete sentences; run-on sentences; and qualifiers.

— Use words which are part of the English language. Do not make up new words.

— Use the professional vocabulary, but consider defining terms which may be unclear.

— Report the facts exactly as they are. Do not make assumptions.

— Become familiar with professional terminology.

— Examine available information and decide what should and should not be included in the report.

— Present ideas and information in logical and/or chronological order.

— Use abbreviations only when they cannot be misinterpreted.

— Use personal pronouns when appropriate.

— Conclude all reports by presenting the names and titles of people who formulated the report. Sign all reports.

If the clinician remembers that a written report is a necessary shortcut for expression of knowledge, the written report can become a basis for making vital decisions. Develop the habit of jotting down brief but concise notes. These notes will serve as valuable firsthand information when writing complete reports. It is the person who can write accurate, clear, concise reports that enjoys an important advantage.

### Questions and Issues

1. Often professionals in Speech Pathology are judged by other professionals according to their report writing skills. Why is this true?

2. There are many different kinds of reports. List the many different kinds of reports that exist and discuss the specific differences and functions of each type of report.

3. Report writing is a simple task and by writing a great number of reports one will become a good report writer. Is the previous statement true or false? Discuss.

4. Why is it necessary to use different terminology to say the same thing when writing different types of reports?

5. Discuss the importance of being specific when writing reports rather than writing in generalities.

# CHAPTER 6

## THE SUPERVISOR–SUPERVISEE CONFERENCE

### Introduction

Michalak (1969) noted that very little is known about the supervisory conference even though this is one of the most frequently employed supervisor techniques utilized by the clinicial supervisor to modify clinical behavior of students. The fact that supervisory conferences are viewed as an important facet of clinical supervision is supported by Schubert and Aitchison (1975). They report that 98 percent of the clinical supervisors used the supervisory conference as an important tool for the supervision and training of student clinicians.

Ward and Webster (1965b) defined clinical supervision as an interactive process between the student and supervisor in which both are working to find productive ways of effecting the diagnostic or therapeutic relationship.

### Function of the Conference

Regardless of which definition one applies to the supervisory conference, the session between the supervisor and clinician should be viewed by the participants as a time for teaching and learning. Of course, the emphasis is upon learning by the student clinician and teaching by the supervisor. However, the supervisor has an opportunity to learn about the clinician. Also, the supervisor can attend to the attitude of the student toward the profession. Likewise, the supervisor may examine the feelings of the clinician regarding the clinical setting and his working with children as opposed to adults. The supervisor is able to become aware of the student's self-evaluation skills, his preference toward therapy procedures, and his knowledge of diagnostic tools.

The supervisor must be alert during the conference and not apply undo pressures which could affect communication between himself and the student. For example, the following comments by the supervisor might represent the truth, but would be better unsaid: "I understand you had difficulty with your supervisor last semester, I'm sure things will be better this semester," "I've heard you aren't very interested in therapy with children," or "I hope you'll take a more sincere interest in your client this semester." There may come a time when the supervisor needs to speak directly to the clinician about the aforementioned topics; but the supervisor should not be "catty." He should be pleasant, honest, and direct, yet diplomatic and to the point.

There is no prescription for how long a supervisory conference should last. The length of the conference is determined by the needs of the clinician and supervisor. Answers to the following questions will determine the approximate length of the conference.

Supervisor related:

— How much information does the supervisor need to supply to the clinician?

— How much information does the supervisor need to obtain from the clinician?

— How much praise and criticism will be provided by the supervisor?

— How direct will the supervisor be in modifying clinician behavior?

— Does the supervisor who is less direct or who is more direct usually require more time for supervisory conferences?

— How much irrelevant information will the supervisor provide?

Clinician related:

— How familiar is the clinician with the client's background and needs?

— Will the clinician understand and accept the recommendations of the supervisor?

— How many and what kinds of requests will the clinician have
of the supervisor?

— Does the clinician feel comfortable with the supervisor?

— What was the satisfaction of the clinician with past supervisory conferences?

Although the length of the supervisory conference will be
determined by such things as the complexity of the speech disorder
of the client, the experience of the clinician, the background of
the supervisor, and relationships established between the clinician,
client, and supervisor, Underwood (1973) found that a high significant correlation existed between a five-minute random segment
of the conference and the entire supervisory conference. This fact
supports information obtained through the use of other observation systems. The information is that people behave in a set
manner and that a representative sample of this behavior, which
reoccurs rapidly, can be obtained.

### Brief Description of the Underwood Category System for Analyzing Supervisor-Clinician Behavior

The *Underwood Category System for Analyzing Supervisor-
Clinician Behavior* was designed to analyze behaviors which occur
between the supervisor and the clinician during the supervisory
conference. The Underwood system is a modification of the
Blumberg system, which has been used to analyze interactions
during supervisory-teacher conferences.

The Underwood system includes a total of seventeen behaviors
to be analyzed during the supervisory conference, nine categories
describing supervisory behavior (1-9) and seven categories describing clinician behavior (10-16). The one remaining category (17)
allows for the recording of silence or confusion.

Each change of behavior which occurs in the conference is
scored using the number which corresponds to the category that
best describes the behavior.

The sixteen behaviors used to analyze supervisor-clinician interaction are:

**Supervisor Behaviors**

1. Supportive
2. Praise
3. Identifies Problem
4. Uses Clinician's Ideas
5. Requests Factual Information
6. Provides Factual Information
7. Requests Opinions and Suggestions
8. Provides Opinions and Suggestions
9. Criticism

**Clinician Behaviors**

10. Identifies Problem
11. Requests Factual Information
12. Provides Factual Information
13. Requests Opinions and Suggestions
14. Provides Opinions and Suggestions
15. Positive Social Behavior
16. Negative Social Behavior

**Supervisor Clinician Behavior**

17.  Silence and Confusion

The specific procedures, methods of analysis and direct application of this system are presented in Underwood (1974).

Using the *Underwood Category System for Analyzing Supervisor-Clinician Behaviors* developed by Underwood (1974), Nelson (1975) examined the frequency of occurrence of behaviors exhibited by supervisors and clinicians during the supervisory conference. The author concluded that during the conference the supervisor used more time talking than did the clinician. In an earlier study, Underwood (1973) concluded that ineffective supervisory conferences, as rated by clinicians and supervisors, were dominated by supervisor talk, while conferences rated as effective showed more clinician talk.

Schubert and Nelson (1976) found that during the supervisory conference the supervisor spends most of his time providing suggestions and opinions about the clinician's therapy behavior. During the supervisory conference the second most frequently occurring behavior used by the supervisor was providing factual information. The supervisor spent sixty-five percent of the time talking; whereas, the clinician spent thirty-five percent of the time talking during the supervisory session.

During the thirty-five percent of the time used by the clinicians in the supervisory conference, the most frequently used behaviors were those of providing suggestions and opinions regarding the therapy session. This behavior was followed by the clinician providing factual information. Although the supervisor dominated the supervisory conference by talking almost twice as much as the clinician, the conferences were rated as effective by both the clinician and the supervisor on independent ratings. The term effective was defined as a good learning experience for improving or modifying therapy behaviors or procedures.

The supervisor should enter the supervisory conference prepared to direct the conference in a manner similar to that which he expects the clinician to use when directing the therapy session. The supervisor needs to be organized and prepared to meet his objectives. The supervisor needs to establish his objectives and then develop procedures for accomplishing the stated objectives. The supervisor should have specific comments and descriptive and objective information to present to the student. The supervisor should know exactly what recommendations he needs to make and then present these recommendations to the clinician in a logical order. When recommendations are made to the clinician, the supervisor should take time to explain why he is making each recommendation and how this recommendation will improve the situation.

The supervisor should be careful in his use of praise. This does not mean that praise should be eliminated; it means that praise should only be given when it is sincere and warranted by the behavior of the clinician.

Simon (1975) notes that it is important for the supervisor to focus or summarize his comments. The author points out that the summary should be concerned with such things as: appropriateness of materials being used, administration and scoring of assessment tools, accuracy of auditory discrimination, methods of motivation, response ratio, rapport maintenance, clarity of directions, and appropriateness of lesson plans and written reports. All of these behaviors are clinician oriented and serve to provide the student clinician with a baseline from which to work.

As the conference draws to a close, the supervisor should consider reviewing the most important aspects of the conference. Reviews should not be automatic with every conference, but should only be conducted when ample time is available and the parties involved are not fatigued.

Before the conference is terminated, it is important that the participants have an opportunity to ask and answer questions. The people involved need to leave the session with a feeling of accomplishment and understanding. Also, the conference should end with both the clinician and supervisor having a clear understanding of future objectives and procedures for accomplishing these objectives.

### Summary

In summary, the supervisory conference is a time for the exchange of ideas and opinions between the supervisor and the clinician. It is a time of teaching and learning by both the clinician and the supervisor. The conference is a time of planning and preparing by the supervisor and clinician to assure the use of appropriate procedures during future therapy sessions.

The supervisory conference is a time for channeling energy for the benefit of the client, clinician, and the supervisor. The supervisory conference should benefit the clinician through improved therapy sessions in the future. The main benefit to the clinician is one of modification and improvement in therapy skills. Finally the supervisor profits from the clinician's feedback. The emphasis of the supervisory conference should not be placed on supervisory improvement; but the supervisor should evaluate himself, as he expects the clinician to self-evaluate the therapy session.

The *Underwood Category System for Analyzing Supervisor-Clinician Behavior* is a useful and necessary tool for analyzing the supervisor-supervisee conference. The system, containing seventeen categories, provides objective and quantifiable information

This kind of information is valuable for improving supervisory skills and for making the conference a more meaningful session. Also, the collected data and information are useful in training clinicial supervisors.

## Questions and Issues

1. How important is the supervisor-supervisee conference to changing the clinical behavior of the student clinician?

2. How often should supervisor-supervisee conferences be held? What are the variables which determine this?

3. What preparation should a supervisor do preceding a conference with a clinician?

4. If an argument emerges between clinician and supervisor, how should the supervisor handle the situation?

5. Discuss and plan for ways of making the supervisor-supervisee conference a meaningful experience.

# CHAPTER 7

## VIDEO TAPE AND CLOSED CIRCUIT TELEVISION

### Introduction

With the increased enrollment in speech pathology programs during the past ten years, problems have evolved. A lack of space is often a problem. A lack of the desired variety of cases is often a concern. But no problem is greater than the lack of adequate supervision.

There are numerous possible reasons for the lack of adequate supervision. One reason is that there is a genuine lack of adequately trained supervisors. Another reason is if adequately trained supervisors are available, they receive a caseload of student clinicians which is too large and, therefore, impossible to supervise adequately. This second point leads us to the discussion of the use of closed circuit television and videotape recording (VTR).

### Advantages

O'Neill and Peterson (1964) suggested the use of the closed circuit television primarily as an instructional tool whereby many clinicians could observe therapy at one time in a class situation. The authors also acknowledged the use of this procedure as an aid to supervision. It is suggested that two or three student clinicians conducting therapy could be monitored in a central control room at one time by one supervisor; thus freeing time which could realistically be used for other supervisory duties, such as conferring and correcting lesson plans.

A second advantage of the use of closed circuit television is the fact that the supervisor does not actually have to be in the room while therapy is in progress. This allows the clinician control of the therapy setting, along with the benefit of the feedback which can be provided following the therapy session.

O'Neill and Peterson further commented that the use of the television camera was neither a major problem nor a distraction after the first few sessions. In fact, the camera is actually an advantage in that close up views which are not possible when viewing through a one-way mirror are possible. The use of closed circuit television in supervision would appear to be of a particular advantage in speech pathology departments where space and/or personnel are limited.

The comments on the use of the closed circuit television for instructional and supervisional purposes were expressed primarily before the advent of popular use of videotape recording. Initially the cost of VTR equipment was prohibitive for many institutions.

Although quite expensive, the advantages of its use appear to balance the cost. Unique situations are captured via television.

## Use of VTR in Supervision

During the late 1960's and early 1970's the use of videotape recording became popular. Some of the uses of a VTR unit are evident. One such use is in supervision. Here, the student-clinician is videotaped for all or part of the therapy session and upon playback of the videotape the clinician is able to self-analyze and the supervisor is able to point out positive and negative behaviors which occurred during the therapy session. The use of the videotape removes the necessity of the supervisor having to recreate through verbal description an occurrence that happened during the therapy session which the supervisor wants to make reference to. Often the clinician will acknowledge a particular situation which the supervisor has recreated when, in reality, the student clinician does not know what the supervisor is talking about. In this instance, the student clinician tries to fake his way through a clinical situation because he believes he should remember the occasion and does not want to appear antagonistic to the supervisor. Also, with the videotape playback, there can be no question as to what behavior did and did not occur. The supervisor can be very specific and point out exactly what he is referring to in each instance.

As mentioned earlier, self-analysis by the student clinician is important as a method of supervision. The student clinician is able to view the videotape and be self-analytical. The student should look for errors which he has made and be willing to point them out to the supervisor when the tape is viewed jointly. The student clinician should seek the supervisor's recommendations. The student clinician should view the tape in an effort to find out which particular behaviors may have led to problem situations. The use of an honest self-viewing and self-analysis of a videotape is extremely valuable. Self-viewing of videotapes can also be done by the student following the viewing of the videotape by the student and the supervisor. At this point, the student clinician should re-examine all the behaviors, good and poor, which were brought to his attention by the supervisor. A mental effort should be made by the student clinician to remove the undesirable behaviors and accent the positive ones.

Videotape recording can be used by the supervisor and student clinician when objective scoring systems are used to quantify the behaviors of the student clinician and client. In fact, with some observation systems it is necessary that videotaping be completed, followed by scoring and analyzing the behaviors from the videotapes. In this way a very accurate count can be obtained of observable behaviors.

By counting behaviors which occurred during a particular session or sessions quantifiable objectives can be established. For example, reinforcers to stimuli can be counted during a therapy session. If the ratio is too low, a measurable objective can be established and examined.

Conferences between the supervisor and student clinician can also be videotaped and observed. This is of particular concern to the supervisor. In this situation the supervisor needs to be self-analytical. He needs to view the tape in an effort to determine what he is doing that appears to excite and motivate the student-clinician. The supervisor needs to observe his own behavior for clues which serve as a deterrent to communication. The following questions should be considered. Is the supervisor pushing his ideas and procedures onto the student clinician before seeking the ideas and thoughts of the student? Is the supervisor overly critical, seldom pointing out the good things the student-clinician has done? In the same manner that the supervisor and student clinician are able to establish behavioral objectives from the videotape for the student clinician, the supervisor can do the same thing concerning his behaviors during the supervisory conference.

Videotape recordings of particular therapy sessions are excellent teaching tools to be used by the supervisor when supervising other student clinicians. Here the supervisor is able to demonstrate, via videotape, behaviors which he hopes to develop and see in student-clinicians. The supervisor is able to view and discuss those behaviors which should not take place.

The supervisor can use, for demonstrative purposes, videotapes of master clinicians. Using this effective method, the student-clinician is able to observe a skilled person applying correct behavioral modification techniques, controlling a hyperactive child, and modifying or changing activities to keep client interest. The supervisor can store and demonstrate clinical activities in a relatively inexpensive manner, and situations which are impossible to recreate in a live session at the exact time desired can also be retained.

Many of the advantages which can be recognized through the use of videotape recording have been pointed out. Along with these advantages, one should note that videotapes can be reused, thereby using the tape again when the information which was initially stored on the tape is no longer useful. Videotape recording can be conducted from outside the therapy room, and possible disruption of therapy does not need to occur. The normal process in this situation would be to have the videotape recorder, camera and tape located in a room adjacent to the therapy room. The two rooms would be separated by a one-way mirror, and recording would be completed in the adjacent room through the one-way mirror.

## Important Non-Supervisory Uses of VTR

Although most videotape recordings pertaining to clinical occurrence might be used by the supervisor at some time, other uses
exist which may not involve the supervisor directly.

First, a library of tapes can be established. These tapes can
then be labeled and used by students and faculty for a variety of
learning experiences. Tapes dealing with cleft palate may be viewed
by a student clinician who has been assigned a cleft palate case. On
the other hand, a faculty member while teaching in the area of cleft
palate may want to show the tape, or at least a segment of the
tape. In a training institution where the type and number of clients
are limited, the tape library is of utmost importance.

Diagnostic sessions can be videotaped for future viewing, evaluation or demonstration purposes. It is obvious that the supervisor
could and may use diagnostic tapes as a teaching tool, but these
tapes may be used in a variety of other ways. If enough tapes are
available, it is a good idea to keep videotapes of diagnostic sessions
for playback and comparison after the client has been in therapy.

Most training institutions are delinquent in an important use
of videotape. That is in making use of the tapes to educate the
parents of the clients. It is possible to have parents view tapes while
a qualified person explains what is being done and why. Improvement in speech patterns can be pointed out and parents can better
understand why and how to complete home speech assignments
made by the clinician. Viewing of videotapes stimulates questions
which parents would have never thought to ask and these questions
help the student-clinician and supervisor to understand and to
work with the client in an improved manner. Having to talk about
and explain things helps the supervisor and clinician to better
understand the client and his parents.

Another area which involves parents and other people who
would be in the waiting room of the speech and hearing clinic is the
use of videotapes to educate these people, in a general sense, about
speech, language, and hearing. Through specially prepared video-

tapes, information can be presented to interested people while they are in the waiting room of the clinic. Tapes can be presented on a great variety of topics. General areas of interest would include normal speech and language development, normal hearing development, pathological conditions related to all areas of speech pathology and audiology, testing and evaluating procedures, normal and abnormal hearing, explanation of an audiogram, purpose and operation of the speech and hearing clinic, the importance of the clinic to the university and community, and perhaps some videotapes concerning the feelings and attitudes of parents who have children with speech disorders.

Videotapes are very useful in the area of research. From videotapes qualitative and quantitative measurements can be made. Videotape recordings provide the researcher with valuable information which cannot be restored in its original form in any other way. The use of videotapes has probably been the single most important development in the area of clinical research in the last ten years.

## Disadvantages of VTR

There are a few disadvantages of videotape recordings which should be mentioned. First, the videotape recording should not be used as a substitute for supervision, but rather they should be used in conjunction with direct supervision and direct feedback. Next the use of videotape recording may be very threatening to the student-clinician. However, in most cases, the student-clinician learns to accept the viewing and reviewing of videotapes as an important, valuable and natural occurrence. Next, the equipment may be distracting to both the student-clinician and supervisor. This is a temporary situation until those concerned become accustomed to the situation.

The last two items to be categorized as disadvantages when using VTR are disadvantages which apply to most kinds of mechanical equipment. Equipment is susceptible to breakdown and, like most pieces of equipment, the videotape equipment always seems to break down when it is most needed. The last item to be mentioned here is the cost and time delay often experienced with videotape equipment. When a piece of equipment wears out or is damaged, it can be extremely expensive to have that piece of equipment repaired or replaced. The possibility of breakdown and damage happening needs to be accounted for within the repair budget.

Whether or not a breakdown creates a dollar and cents problem, it may cause a lengthy delay in the use of the equipment. Sometimes it is possible to cope with a delay by borrowing equipment which can be used during some of the time your own equipment is incapacitated. Each professional setting needs to handle the situation as best it can with the available resources.

## Summary

The use of videotape recordings as a method of supervising student clinicians is invaluable. Recording provides a reliable storage of information until the supervisor and/or student-clinician has an opportunity to view the tape. Videotape recording provides direct and exact feedback to the student-clinicians. From recordings, behaviors can be quantified and qualified, thereby videotapes provide a method of analyzing changes in clinical behaviors of both the student clinician and the client.

Videotape recording should be viewed by the clinical supervisor in an effort to improve his supervisory behaviors. Self-analysis and self-improvement is as important to the supervisor as the same items are to the student-clinician concerning his clinical behaviors.

Videotapes store important clinical information which can be used for demonstration purposes for students, faculty, parents, and other interested people. Effort should be made to make maximal use of videotape library materials. Also, an effort should be made to stock and label a speech, language, and hearing videotape library.

Videotapes can be shown to parents and relatives of children who have a speech disorder in an effort to help these people understand more fully the problem and the difficulties associated with the treatment. Such things as hypertensive behavior and lack of motivation can be demonstrated to viewers.

The use of videotapes for research purposes in the area of clinical supervision and treatment of clients should not be over-looked. It is only through continued investigation in these areas that we are able to improve our services. Research and service are hand-in-hand products and should not be viewed as dichoto-mous.

The few areas which can be presented as disadvantageous when using videotape recordings need to be coped with. Disadvan-tages in using videotape equipment are present, as they are with most forms of equipment. The main concern when using video equipment is the susceptibility to breakdown. The supervisor must not become overly dependent on using this equipment. In conjunction with breakdown of equipment the concern is for the cost of repairs. This is a natural phenomenon, as is breakdown, and the users of videotape equipment must learn to cope with both factors.

## Questions and Issues

1. List and discuss the assets of using videotape recording as part of the clinical training program.

2. Explain the difference between closed circuit television and videotape recordings. When is closed circuit television more valuable than videotape recordings?

3. Can videotape recordings be used as part of the student's self-evaluation program? If so, how can videotape recordings be used to their maximum potential?

4. List and explain as many uses as you can for videotape re-cordings in a clinical training program.

5. Investigate the total cost of obtaining and maintaining an adequate videotape recording system in your clinical program.

# CHAPTER 8

## NONVERBAL COMMUNICATION

### Introduction and Definition

Communication includes all of the processes by which one individual may affect another. Verbal communication, which is only one aspect of the total communication process, is a specific form of message transmission which uses word symbols to represent real objects and ideas. The counterpart of verbal communication is nonverbal communication. The human body is continually sending out messages. These messages are interpreted by the observers before they hear the verbal message. Signals are sent out by every part of our bodies: the hands, the face, the head, the shoulders, the fingers, the legs, the torso of the body, and the feet. In everyday conversations we make many important judgments and decisions based on nonverbal cues. Much nonverbal communication is involuntary and is not consciously controlled. Thus, much communication via the nonverbal behavior of an individual occurs while the person is unaware that a message is being transmitted. It is impossible for us to turn off our bodies and not transmit a message about ourselves. Egolf and Chester (1973) point out that it is impossible to have social contact without transmission of nonverbal cues.

Nonverbal communication contributes significantly to human communication. What the receiver of a message sees plays a very important role in his interpretation of what the sender is saying. Usually the receiver of a communication interprets the nonverbal signal as being more important than the verbal signal. As the time-worn saying goes, "Actions speak louder than words." To illustrate, consider the case in the 1968 Olympic games when several Black athletes wore the black arm bands and raised clenched fists as they were presented their medals. Not a word was spoken, but the entire world felt the impact. The athletes were booed during the games as they were spectators as well as competitors and were publicly disgraced. While this was occurring, George Foreman, another Black athlete, was winning the Gold Medal in boxing. When he was presented his medal, the arm band of black was obviously missing. And, as the others had raised clenched fists, he, instead, raised a small American flag. He became an instant hero; not only to those who were Olympic game fans, but to the patriotic American. Again, no words were spoken. It was in actions, gestures, body movements and facial expressions that these men, all winners in the Olympic games, became heroes and villains.

The sender, too, relies on visual cues sent to him from the receiver to indicate the impact of his message. In normal communication, the verbal components carry less than thirty-five percent of the social meaning of a situation, whereas sixty-five percent of the meaning is conveyed with nonverbal cues. If a person desires to prove to himself the value of nonverbal communication, all that he needs to do is walk down the street and smile a greeting or wave the hand. These nonverbal cues are answered immediately. It is difficult not to respond to a smile with a smile. This is something that all persons respond to.

In speech pathology and particularly in the clinical setting where emphasis is on the effectiveness of communication, nonverbal communication is a valuable part of sending messages. Egolf and Chester (1973) point out that nonverbal behavior should be of particular concern to those people associated with normal and pathological human interaction.

### Environmental and Cultural Nonverbal Behaviors

Many nonverbal behaviors occur because of the environmental and cultural patterns. Many studies have shown that the size of the room and the placement of the furniture have determined the success or failure of a meeting. A clinician should be aware of the beliefs and attitudes of an individual so that misunderstandings do not occur. For example, in certain cultures the shape of the table is important. Round tables are used if all members are equal; rec-

tangular tables are used when there is a leader and several subordi-
nate positions involved in a decision making process. In this instance, severe communication barriers may be established and communication, regardless of the fact that it is well planned, will not
occur or will be severely interrupted.

In many cultures, the seating arrangements determine the communication pattern. The Oriental race, as well as the American
Indian, place much emphasis on personal arrangements in a conversational or a communicational situation. In addition to the placement of an individual, the conversational distance must also be a
factor during communication. Americans, as well as other nation-
alities, have established conversational norms which are very important to the success of a communication situation. One of the
norms of concern is the distance between the communication participants. If one member stands too close, a barrier to communication is established; however, if the communicator stands or sits too
far away, communication breaks down, also. The Arabs and South
Americans stand or sit very close together when they communicate.
In fact, the breath of the person sending the message can almost
be felt. However, the Germans stand at some distance as they
communicate. An interesting experience is to observe the habits
of clerks in department stores and try to determine their environmental or cultural heritage as they help the customers. If a person
is of a proud or humble culture, this will undoubtedly come through
in their selling situation. If a race or nationality of people feels
humble, the clerk will stand near the person and try to establish a
communicational situation which is desirable. On the other hand,
if the clerk feels superior to the customer, he will keep the counter
between them and discontinue the communicational situation
quickly. Often this breakdown in communication is termed rude
or poor salesmanship. Nevertheless, it occurs and should be recognized. The clinician must realize this situation might occur in the
clinical situation. Some communicational breakdowns may occur
when the clinician sits on one side of the table and the client on
the other. Or, communication may be more successful if the client
and the clinician sit side by side.

As this personal distance norm is considered, the personal space norm can be included. All humans have their own personal space and if this space is trespassed upon, they are offended. For example, when eating at a restaurant, each place is set usually with the help of a placemat or a table setting pattern. This placemat or table setting silently says, "This is your place. No one else can interfere." If anyone reaches over and helps himself to your water or your cup, you immediately speak or act in such a way that they are much aware that they have violated your personal space. The same thing is true in the clinical situation. The clinician places the materials and supplies for the session in such a manner that they silently say, "These are yours. These are mine." The client uses only those things designated his. When personal space is violated, the communication participants are offended and communication barriers are set up or communication breaks down entirely.

As the space norms exist, it must be noted that seating arrangements determine the kind of work which will occur. For instance, if the participants are seated across from each other they work individually but share ideas. If the participants sit side-by-side, they work cooperatively. The results of their effort are obtained from both working together toward one goal. And, if the participants sit diagonally, they work competitively and independently.

One more norm to consider concerning cultural influences is that of personal contact or touch. Some cultures consider personal contact or touch very necessary for communication while others feel it taboo to have personal contact. Again, there have been studies directed toward personal contact. Jourard (1966) performed a study where he watched couples in a restaurant in San Juan, Puerto Rico; Paris, France; Gainsville, Florida; and London, England. He counted the number of times these couples touched. The results were interesting. The couple he observed in Puerto Rico touched 180 times in one hour. The couple in Paris touched 110 times in one hour. The couple in Gainsville touched two times and the couple in London did not touch at all in one hour. From this study it can be assumed that touch is more important to some than it is to others. Also, it is accepted by some and not by others. Some children, as well as adults, respond favorably to a literal pat on the back, while others react negatively to any such overture. Some clinicians may find that by placing a hand lightly on the shoulder or around the shoulder the communication situation will be pleasant. With some children, the clinician may find that touch is frightening or that the child will pull away from touch in any form.

The cultural and environmental heritage of individuals may help to determine the success or failure of the clinical therapy situation. No one can say this is an absolute cause for success or failure. One can only suggest that the clinician and supervisor be aware that these factors do exist and that they may be an influence. Not only may they affect the child in the therapy session, but they might create communication barriers between the clinician and the parents. The parents may become offended and withdrawn so they do not communicate needed background information nor volunteer information as to the progression of the client in his everyday behaviors.

### Positive and Negative Nonverbal Behaviors

Especially important in the clinical setting are those nonverbal behaviors which serve as stimuli and reinforcers, both positive and negative. These valuable nonverbal cues are important for behavior modification.

The positive nonverbal behaviors which are most important to the clinician and supervisor are: eye contact, smile, positive head nod, gesture, positive touch, postural change, forward lean, facial expressions, dress, and tone of voice. Following is a discussion of each of these nonverbal behaviors.

### Eye Contact:

Eye contact is defined as looking in the direction of the face of the person with whom one is communicating or with whom one is attempting to communicate. Eye contact plays an important role in communicating interpersonal attitudes and in establishing rela-tionships. Eye control in a normal situation cannot be controlled easily. The eyes can show emotions clearly. Eye contact can cause anxiety if it is absent or if the contact is of long duration and it becomes a stare. If a person wants to avoid the situation, then eye contact is avoided in the communication. When eye contact is missing, the communication is affected. Eye contact is used as a signal in initiating encounters, in greetings, as a reinforcer, and to indicate that a point of view has been understood. Mehrabian and Williams (1969) demonstrated that increasing degrees of persuasive effort were associated with increase in eye contact with the addressee. Eye contact is a spontaneous reaction and, as such, is particularly useful to the clinician and supervisor during the initial interview session and during subsequent conversational periods. Eye contact is useful when trying to persuade. In fact, studies have shown that facial expression including eye contact was generally more effective than the vocal channel.

*Smile:*

The extension of the lips in a bilateral direction defines a smile. The smile is only one part of the facial expression that contributes to the total communication act. The smile is an adaptive movement of the person responding to internal and external stimuli. It, too, is a spontaneous reaction and as such has an immediate impact on the communication situation. A smile is contagious. It is usually interpreted as having a pleasant meaning. As mentioned earlier in the chapter, a smile can be a greeting or a pleasing gesture of friendship. It is difficult not to respond to a smile. The smile is an immediate reward and, as such, is a useful tool to the clinician. A child responds to a smile in much the same way an adult responds to a verbal compliment. Mehrabian and Williams (1969) found that the rate of smiling reflected liking of the addressee. Higher rates of smiling indicate greater efforts of the communicator to relieve tension and discomfort.

*Positive Touch:*

Touch of a positive nature is defined as bodily contact between people other than to restrain or punish. Touch in this case is reinforcing or instructional. Bordeen (1971) had a subject interact with another person under three conditions: touching only, visual only, and verbal only. The touch encounters were described by the participants as trustful, sensitive, natural, mature, serious, and warm.

Mehrabian (1969) found touching to be associated with a positive attitude. Touch is a nonverbal behavior which can be more successful with children than with adults. Children appear to respond to the friendly touch. Possibly this goes back to the tender loving care and caressing given to the child as an infant. The warmth of the touch can improve a communication session. It must be remembered, however, that as the child grows older he becomes more inhibited and more aware of touch. In a study on touch by Jourard (1966), the following observations were found to be significant. Jourard questioned students regarding the parts of the human body which they felt were accessible touch areas. He included touching by mother, father, friends of the same sex, and friends of the opposite sex. His findings were that females were considerably more accessible to touch than were the males.

As one considers whether or not touch should be used, the individual must be considered. The environment of the child determines in large part what will be successful and what will ultimately end in failure. Some children do not accept touch as sincere and friendly because all the touch that they have experienced has been performed in hate and meanness. When a child withdraws from touch, the clinician should become concerned. This may stem from experiences which have caused other problems in the therapy session. Studies show that children who were deprived of handling and mothering as infants are prone to show difficulties in reading and speech. Sometimes these deprived children seem retarded in their development. It usually is not retardation, but confusion in tactile communication. Touch is a crucial part of human communication.

Children seem to thrill and respond if they are treated like adults. Handshaking, an example of a touching behavior, exemplifies this fact. Children enjoy shaking hands. They have seen adults shaking hands or they have seen well-known people whom they admire greet each other in a manner using the tactile sense. To them, if you extend this greeting, you are trying to be friendly and they will usually react satisfactorily.

*Positive Head Nod:*

A movement of the head in a distinct back and forth direction on a vertical plane defines positive head nod. In a study completed by Rosenfield (1966), it was found head nods correlated with smiles and both acted as reinforcers. Positive head nods signal continued interest and attention to the speaker.

Dittman and Llewellyn (1968) stated that from their study they found head nods are most likely to be observed at points of interaction between speaker and listener; therefore, head nods have a social function. The clinician may encourage the client to respond with a nod of the head. Often, games children play and enjoy involve the nodding of the head. Children see this behavior occur from infancy on and they respond because they remember that this behavior resulted in being liked.

In addition to being a conditioned response, the nodding of the head as someone either initiates an idea or responds to an idea seems to be a natural reflex. Natural behaviors often create a feeling of friendship and sincerity; therefore, they should be used in the clinical setting as often as is necessary to create a friendly atmosphere.

*Gestures:*

A gesture is defined as a movement of the arm, hand, or finger which is not in moving contact with another part of the body. However, the definition of gesturing should not stop there. It should include not only the hand but other parts of the body, too. The head can gesture, legs and feet can gesture, and so can the torso of the body. For the purpose of simplicity, the author has included nodding the head and positive changes of the body in separate sections of this chapter. Examples of gestures which will be included here are pointing, clapping, illustrating, defining, or commanding gestures, i.e., "over there," "sit here," "see this." Gesturing is almost as common in human interaction as oral communication. Frequently gesturing is coordinated with speaking, but it is fully possible and probable that we gesture when we do not speak. Persons speak less than they gesture because they can gesture as they listen as well as when they speak. Some gestures are so common to humans that no verbal message needs to accompany the gesture; however, a gesture and a verbal message must agree or confusion exists. The clinician must recognize when the child is confused by gestures. For example, when clapping is used, the child must understand that it is part of a game or of the therapy exercise or he may confuse it with clapping done by a parent to command. When confusion is present, the child cannot respond as expected.

Gesturing has replaced verbal explanation in several instances. One gesture can be used instead of loaded words or words with double meanings. When a clinician indicates to a child to place a mark "there," it is easier to point and show the child rather than give the child a verbal direction which might be confusing.

Gesturing can be ambiguous and cause several communication problems. One of the most confusing gestures is the "V" sign. This can be a sign of peace or greeting. Depending upon the cultural background, the understanding of this sign can have more or fewer implications than is actually meant. It can also mean the number two.

Studies have shown that when a person is trying to persuade, he uses many more gestures than he uses in a situation where persuasion is not a prime objective. As the clinician persuades the client to respond, he will undoubtedly use many gestures. This might also indicate that the clinician is attempting to build up a friendship with the client. Studies have shown that relationships are strengthened by gestures. Mehrabian (1968a) stated that greater liking is conveyed by using gestures.

*Postural Change and Forward Lean:*

A postural change is defined as a gross movement of the body trunk (torso) or shift in position of the hips. Forward lean is a forward movement of the upper body, taking place at the level of the hips. Mehrabian (1968a, 1969) found that a forward lean toward the addressee resulting in a smaller distance between communicator and addressee indicated a more positive attitude. Mehrabian also pointed out that distinctive postures were adapted for friendly, hostile, superior, and inferior attitudes. In other research, postural shift was discovered to be meaningful communication and not random acts. In each instance, the position of the body had specific communicative value. In some instances the body moves toward the center of communication and at other times the body moves away from the communicator. Studies showed that when a person liked the communicator, the tendency was to turn toward the communicator with shoulders and torso. Likewise, if a disliking existed between the listener and the speaker, the listener would turn shoulders and torso away from the communicator. In any group discussion there are certain movements worth observing or watching for. Movements such as crossing the arms, crossing the legs, turning the body toward or away from the speaker, leaning the body back or forward, drooping shoulders, and position of the arms either crossed in front of the person or hands placed on the hips indicate the attitude of the person involved. If the clinician observes a lot of body movement, it is an indicator that the client might be bored and maybe the session should be modified or the materials varied. If a client crosses his arms, this may indicate his withdrawal from any further cooperation with the clinician. As clinical session progresses, the clinician should note the client's leaning into or away from therapy. These body positions are strong indicators of interest and attitude.

The counterparts to the positive nonverbal cues, which are frequently used by both the clinician and the supervisor, are negative head nods, frowns, and self-manipulation. The definitions for the negative head nod and the frown include physiological and psychological meanings that would be the opposite of positive head nod and smile. Self-manipulation is defined as a response that involves motion of a part of the body in contact with another part, either directly or mediated by an instrument. Self-manipulation was found to be unrelated to approval-seeking behavior (Rosenfeld, 1966).

### Nonverbal Behaviors Which Accompany Anxieties

There are some specific cues which clinical researchers have identified that accompany specific anxieties and emotions. Before examining some of these cues, the reader should be cautioned that careless generalizations might be misleading. Nevertheless, the significance of the findings are worth mentioning and discussing. One client was observed to cover her eyes with her hand when she discussed things that she was ashamed of; another client would clasp and unclasp his hands when questioned about unfamiliar or unpleasant topics; clients were observed to play with objects or apparel or decorations such as buttons, bracelets, rings, or belts during questioning; scratching was associated with self-attack; the twisting of hair or hands was observed as a gesture of nervous tension; and a client would turn his head to the side as he was confronted with unpleasant stimuli. These are only a few of the specific cues which can be observed as a clinician encounters a client who has a tendency to hesitate or not respond to therapy. A client may need to feel comfortable with the clinician before sharing ideas and before this occurs discomfort may be expressed in one way or another. Self-manipulation is a fairly certain indication that nervous tension exists. Krout (1954) found that there were approximately 5000 distinct hand gestures which indicated anxiety. Just a few of the identified gestures were: movement of the hand to the nose when fear is present; making a fist when aggression is felt; placing the fingers to the lip if shame is to be represented; and frustration is shown by an open hand dangling between one's leg.

## Recent Research

In one of the few studies investigating nonverbal behaviors of student clinicians, Schubert and Mercer (1975) examined the use of nonverbal cues used by student clinicians. The researchers compared the frequency of ten nonverbal cues used by two groups of student clinicians: one group of clinicians was ranked high by supervisors on their personal evaluation, and one group of clinicians was ranked low by supervisors on their personal evaluation. The two groups of clinicians were observed according to the frequency of usage of the following ten nonverbal cues: smile, positive head nod, negative head nod, gesture, self-manipulation, negative touch, positive touch, eye contact, postural change and forward lean. The researchers found that clinicians who were rated high by their supervisors used smiles, positive head nods and eye contact much more frequently than did the clinicians who were rated low. When examining the total use of nonverbal behaviors used by the two groups of clinicians, it was determined that the high-rated clinicians used more nonverbal behaviors than the other group. Student clinicians who were rated low by the supervisor were found to use more distracting self-manipulations during the therapy session than the high-rated clinicians.

In other recent research, Stevens (1976) examined eleven nonverbal behaviors exhibited by two groups of students involved in clinical practicum, beginning student clinicians and advanced student clinicians. The eleven nonverbal behaviors which were noted and studied were: the smile, frown, positive head nod, negative head nod, gestures, self-manipulation, positive touch, negative touch, eye contact, postural change, and forward lean. The researcher studied these behaviors by noting the number of times they occurred during a clinical session. The results indicated that during the actual clinical period the advanced student clinicians and the beginning student clinicians differed in the usage of the eleven nonverbal behaviors. It was found that the advanced student clinicians used the social reinforcing behaviors more often than did the beginning student clinicians. Stevens classified the social reinforcing behaviors as the smile, positive head nod, eye contact, positive touch, and forward lean. The nonverbal behaviors which were classified by Stevens as being undesirable were self-manipulation, postural change, negative head nod, frown, and negative touch. These behaviors were exhibited more often by the beginning student clinicians. The behavior noted most often during the recorded therapy sessions was eye contact and it was used by both groups of student clinicians.

Three groups of student clinicians were studied by Schubert and Gudmundson (1976) to examine the feasibility of teaching nonverbal skills to student clinicians. The researchers matched clinicians in all three groups according to practicum hours completed removing the variance of clinical experience among the subjects. The clinicians studied were divided into three equal groups. Group I received training via videotape playback and verbal instruction.

Group II received verbal instruction only and Group III served as the control group, receiving no videotape nor verbal instruction relating to nonverbal behaviors.

The results of the study showed that Group I increased their use of the nonverbal behaviors eye contact, smile, and negative head nod significantly, while the nonverbal behavior of self-manipulation was decreased significantly. Very little change was noted in either of the remaining two groups. Group II which received verbal instruction only and Group III which received no instruction. In summary, the study points out that the frequency of usage of nonverbal behaviors as used by student clinicians can be changed through instruction and that instruction using videotapes and verbal comments pertaining to nonverbal behaviors produces meaningful results.

## Importance

Children and adults attend to and use nonverbal cues. The clinician must use common sense in the selection of his cues. For example, it doesn't make sense to ruffle up the hair of a 60 year old woman, but this behavior with a five year old boy is likely to be interpreted as a very friendly behavior and at times it may serve as a reinforcer. Whereas, a five year old may not attend to a shift in posture; an adult may interpret a speaker's postural shift as an indication that the speaker has finished speaking. Maintaining a particular posture when speaking indicates a desire to continue to speak.

Following is a list of nonverbal behaviors that the clinician and supervisor should be aware of. Supervisors should observe the use of these behaviors by the clinician. Upon self-evaluation, the clinician needs to be aware of the use and the lack of these behaviors:

— Attend to the person who is speaking to you. It makes the person feel what he is saying is important and that he is important to you as a person. Learning to listen attentively is a skill. An effective listener is able to provide appropriate feedback.

— Look directly at a person when beginning to speak to him. This creates a feeling of openness.

— Keep an average amount of eye contact; look at the person you are speaking to, but don't stare.

— Do smile; this implies satisfaction and a signal to continue.

— Do use your hands; you may imply happiness and satisfaction by clapping. You may hold up your hand to signal a person to wait or stop.

— Do use your fingers to point. Pointing can serve as a correcting signal, a distracting signal, and a stimulus.

— Do change postural position; a forward lean indicates an interest in the other person.

— Do place your hand on the speaker's shoulder, arm, or hand to indicate you desire silence or to improve communication.

The above behaviors can and should be used by the clinician and supervisor to convey more effectively the desired message.

Negative types of nonverbal behaviors can also be used to help convey the message. Examples and the meanings of some negative behaviors include the crossing of the arms on the chest, which is usually viewed as defensive and indicates a closed type of attitude; the hand closed in a fist-like position indicates tension; a person sittting with his legs crossed and one leg in a kicking motion is usually bored or preoccupied with another matter; lowering of the eyebrows which is part of frowning implies disbelief and dissatisfaction. This behavior is one of the most useful and clearly understood negative behaviors a clinician can use. It is often accompanied by a slight turning of the head and is interpreted by the viewer as, "I've made a mistake," or "He disagrees with me," or "I better try another response."

The clinician who is not making full use of nonverbal cues should be made aware of this situation by the supervisor. This means that the supervisor must make every effort to observe and to record the frequencies of these behaviors used by the clinician. Also, the clinician must watch for the use and nonuse of these behaviors when viewing videotapes and doing any type of self-evaluation.

Negative nonverbal cues can be as important as the positive cues. The clinician should use the negative nonverbal cues along with the verbal message to signal the client when an error has been made. Too often, especially with beginning clinicians, errors of the client are not detected, or if the clinician does detect the error, he is unprepared to notify the client. It is imperative that such behaviors be drawn to the attention of the student clinician by the supervisor.

What we do and how we do it is more important than what we say. This statement has been printed and said many times. It could not be truer for any group of people than those classified as speech handicapped. The hard-of-hearing child, the stuttering teenager, and the aphasic adult learn very rapidly to attend to nonverbal cues.

## Summary

Everyone is constantly using nonverbal cues even though they may not be aware of it. Nonverbal cues contribute significantly to the communication process and these cues are valuable to both the sender and receiver of a message.

The important positive nonverbal behaviors which should be part of the clinician's repertoire are: eye contact, smile, positive head nod, gesture, positive touch, postural change, and forward lean. The negative nonverbal behaviors which professionals need to recognize in the professional setting are negative head nod, frown, and self-manipulation. It is imperative that both positive and negative nonverbal cues be used regularly and appropriately by the clinician and supervisor.

Research in the area of speech pathology shows that clinicians who are rated high by supervisors use more nonverbal cues than student clinicians who are rated low. Research also shows that advanced student clinicians use more positive nonverbal behaviors than do the beginning student clinicians. Also the beginning student clinician exhibits more of the nonverbal behaviors classified as undesirable.

Additional research indicates that nonverbal behavioral skills such as eye contact, smiles, and negative head nods can be taught to student clinicians by using the videotape playback and verbal instruction. The implication is that supervisors should be aware of nonverbal cues used and those not used by clinicians. Also, the supervisor must examine the appropriateness of nonverbal cues used by clinicians.

It is apparent from these studies and studies from numerous professions that the use of nonverbal behaviors influence the efficiency of communication. Supervisors should attend to the nonverbal behaviors of the clinicians. The use of nonverbal behaviors by clinicians is related to the overall clinical performance.

## Questions and Issues

1. Explain how nonverbal communication influences the therapy session.

2. What are some nonverbal behaviors which are unique to particular cultures? Why is it that these behaviors have been preserved for hundreds of years?

3. What nonverbal behaviors are of most importance to the clinician in the therapy session? What behaviors are of least value?

4. Explain what is meant by negative nonverbal cues. How does the use of these cues assist the clinician to meet his therapy objectives?

5. Can the use of nonverbal cues be taught to student clinicians? If so, how and when should this be done?

# CHAPTER 9

## SUPPORTIVE PERSONNEL

## IN SPEECH PATHOLOGY

### Introduction

Because the clinical supervisor has such an encompassing responsibility, it is necessary that this person be aware of the potential use, guidelines, and training recommendations related to a group of active people in the profession of Speech Pathology and Audiology referred to by many titles: communication aides, supportive personnel , technicians, nonprofessionals, and para-professionals. This chapter will deal with information concerning aides of which a supervisor should be aware. The chapter also includes information which can be applied directly to the task of preparing clinicians.

The supervisor should make the student clinicians aware that they may be employed in a setting which uses communication aides. Therefore, the student clinician should be familiar with some of the assets and liabilities of a program which employs such aides.

### Purpose of Communication Aides

The purpose of the aide is simple; it is to reduce the time and effort of the professional in administering minimal tasks so that the clinician can increase and intensify his efforts with the more complex communicative disordered person. The communication aide can perform routine tasks which before were the responsibility and time consuming function of the clinician. The communication aide, by assuming the responsibility of completing minimal tasks, helps the professional provide more time for more direct therapy to more people who need the service. Aides also help to decrease the manpower shortage in programs by providing additional services when funds for professional personnel are unavailable.

Communication aides are used in many different ways. Their roles are usually determined by the needs of the employing institutions. However, guidelines have recently been established regarding the function of communication aides.

## Questions Related to Communication Aides

Before examining the specific guidelines pertaining to communication aides, an analysis of some of the concerns relating to the topic of communication aides is in order. Irwin (1967) raised questions some of which are still being asked and answered today. Some of these questions include: Should aides be paid or should they be volunteers? Should aides be of a particular age group? Should aides be trained for the profession? If aides are trained, how specific should the training be? Should aides be licensed? If aides provide therapeutic service, to what degree can this be done? Irwin was also concerned about establishing a reasonable ratio between the number of supportive workers and the number of professional workers.

## Guidelines and Supervision of Communication Aides

The many aspects of supervision regarding aides has been and continues to be a concern. In the past, the general pattern was one of minimal supervision for aides. Often, both the professional and the aide would be scheduled to work with different clients or engaging in different tasks at the same time. Therefore, aides had limited time to observe the professional and the professional had little time to observe the aide.

Because of the early problems concerning communication aides, it was necessary that guidelines be established. In 1970, the American Speech and Hearing Association approved and published the "Guidelines of the Role, Training, and Supervision of the Communication Aide." The guidelines were developed with a task oriented model. These guidelines were devised to provide some type of quality control for those institutions which were planning on using communication aides. Following is a summary of the major points presented in the guidelines (Moncur, 1970).

### The Role and Tasks of the Aide:

— Clinicians with the Certificate of Clinical Competence are responsible to the client for services provided by the aide.

— Decisions in regard to diagnosis, management and future disposition of clients should not be the responsibility of the aides.

— Aides must be adequately trained and qualified to perform the duties required of them.

— The supervising clinician must fully define and delineate the aide's roles and tasks.

— In hiring the speech aides, fair employment practices and general employment requirements should be considered in addition to the following: The aides should possess empathy, an ability to communicate effectively with adults and children, and an ability to understand the cultural and linguistic heritages of the clients.

### Training of the Aides:

— Training should be dictated by the tasks to be performed. (Training in clerical duties and other related tasks do not require policy statements by the American Speech and Hearing Association, ASHA).

— A professional in the specific speech and hearing program should select the aides on the basis of the mental, physical and emotional qualifications necessary to perform the required duties. Appropriate personnel in speech and hearing programs should train the new aides, and aides which have had experience should have the opportunity to be involved in inservice programs.

— On-the-job training should vary depending upon the nature of the work performed and this training should be the responsibility of the organization.

— All training should be provided solely by speech pathologists and audiologists who hold the Certificate of Clinical Competence.

— In-service training and encouragement for self-improvement must be provided to the aides by the employing organization.

— Training must be task-oriented and will vary according to the required task.

— The aides' language, speech, reading, writing, work habits, and professional decorum may require improvement through counseling and guidance.

*Policies and Guidelines Regarding the Direction of Aides:*

— Aides should only work in speech and hearing diagnosis and treatment with the direction of an ASHA member holding the Certificate of Clinical Competence.

— The clients' welfare is the legal, ethical, and moral responsibility of the ASHA certified directors under which the aides work.

*Guidelines for the Clinician Include:*

— A qualified professional must initially evaluate each client.

— It is the clinician's responsibility to outline and direct the specific program for clinical management.

— Direct contact by the clinician with the client must be maintained throughout the course of therapy.

— The case must be reviewed by the supervising clinician at the termination of therapy.

— Clinical services provided by the aides must be terminated if conditions prevent the above guidelines from being followed.

*Administration:*

— This committee strongly recommends that service programs which employed aides be registered by the Professional Services Board of Examiners in Speech Pathology and Audiology.

— Direction which is provided to the aides must preclude independence in clinical decision-making.

— The program director is responsible for insuring that the above guidelines are met. The recommended ratio of communication aides to certified professionals should be four to one.

The guidelines, although providing initial guidance concerning supportive personnel, did not specify requirements for supervision, other than requiring the supervisor to have the Certificate of Clinical Competence (CCC) issued by the American Speech and Hearing Association. As discussed by Culatta, Colucci, and Wiggins (1975), many supervisors holding the Certificate of Clinical Competence did not view the certificate as a valid criterion for assessing supervisory competence. Other professionals have also stressed the importance of requiring minimal standards for supervision beyond the Certificate of Clinical Competence. Nelson (1973) noted the importance of internship experience in the area of supervision and Schubert (1974b) suggested that minimal standards be established for persons in supervisory positions.

## Qualities and Training of Paraprofessionals

It is impossible to present all of the possible qualities a communication aide should have. It is just as impossible to present all of the information the technician should have regarding his training as an aide. Each individual and distinct setting is unique, and it is necessary to select people, as best one can, for the particular position in a specific location. Selection criteria must be established for the particular job and available personnel.

In a large metropolitan area, a minimum of two years of college might be established as a minimum requirement for a communication aide; whereas in a rural area a high school diploma may be too rigid of a requirement. Whatever the education or age of the communication aide may be, the following is a list of qualities the aide should meet:

— Be old enough and mature enough to understand the communication problems of children and adults

— Be able to communicate effectively

— Be cooperative and dependable

— Be energetic

— Have empathy for people

— Have sympathy for people

— Have a desire to want to help people who have a communication disorder

— Have normal speech and hearing

The training programs concerning communication aides must be directed toward the specific task the aide will be asked to perform. This does not mean that, if time allows, general background information regarding the profession of Speech Pathology and Audiology should not be provided. In fact, this would be ideal but is often impractical.

Some of the areas for discussion or direct training topics which the aide should be involved in are as follows:

— The speech and hearing mechanism

— The duties and responsibilities of the clinician

— The duties and responsibilities of the communication aide

— Ethical conduct

— Normal speech, language and hearing

— Abnormal speech, language and hearing

— Therapy procedures

— Establishing therapy objectives

— Evaluating therapy behavior

— Use of operant procedures in therapy

— Phonetics and phonology

— Clerical responsibilities

Again, it is important to stress that all of the above listed areas do not need to be included as part of the aide's training. The emphasis of the training must be in the area in which the person is to function. For example, if the aide is to administer articulation therapy using operant procedures, then the training needs to accent phonetics, articulation therapy, and the use of operant procedures.

## Problems Relating to Communication Aides

Educational variability of aides can be a problem. Some aides with several years of college education feel they are as well informed as their supervisors. This leads to the question as to whether professionally qualified persons should be employed as technicians, and if they are what regulations need to be applied. Schubert (1974c) suggests that professionals take a position on the use of qualified and certified teachers being employed as aides. He suggested that aides should be paid according to their qualifications and offered the following points in support of that position.

1. A certified clinician has devoted much time and energy to his preparation and should not be taken advantage of by economic circumstances beyond his control.

2. The certified clinician serving as a communication aide is as well qualified as the regular clinician and should not be paid less than half (any fraction) of what the regular teacher receives for the same number of hours worked. The communication aide should be paid according to his qualifications.

3. Often the certified clinician serving as a communication aide is performing professional tasks.

4. Certified clinicians in some school systems feel they must work a year or two as an aide before they will be considered seriously as a prospect for a regular clinical position.

The problem of too little and too much education is of prevalent concern. The need for education must be determined by the tasks to be provided by the communication aide. It is important that a specific job description be completed for each aide position.

If the aide has better therapy ideas and techniques than the supervisor, this causes feelings of inadequacy and jealousy within the supervisor. When this happens, it is likely that the supervisor will be antagonized by the aide, resulting in a strained relationship.

There exists a concern by professionals that they may be replaced by the aide who is not as well educated, and who will work for a lower salary. Negative attitudes toward the employment of communication aides center around the idea of many participating and non-participating clinicians that their jobs might be in jeopardy.

Many clinicians and other professionals doubt the effectiveness of aides due to their lack of training and experience. This condition leads to a lack of cooperation by professionals who believe they are wasting their time and that the aide is serving as a hindrance toward improving the communicative problem of the client.

Also, some clinicians feel that their role will change from that of providing treatment to that of being a diagnostician. The clinicians are concerned that the aide will provide treatment to too many clients and the clinician will be assigned to evaluation tasks and working only with problem cases.

The supervision and training of aides is of the utmost concern. It is imperative that the employing agency has appropriate reasons for hiring aides. When the reasons for employing aides are meaningful and well established, then one knows the purpose in training the aides. Proper supervision must be given to the aides by certified, knowledgeable, and experienced supervisors. Therefore, time must be allowed for the supervisor to complete the necessary task of guiding and advising the communication aide.

## Success of Programs Using Aides

Research conducted in the use of communication aides has included studies on the abilities of aides to detect speech problems and conduct therapy for specified speech problems. Klinkhammer (1966) supported the use of nonprofessionals in the school systems. The author reported that in Maryland every local school system employed nonprofessionals in their special education program in one capacity or another. He also noted that the use of nonprofessionals resulted in the improvement of services both qualitatively and quantitatively to children.

In an investigation conducted by Ham (1968) it was found that children with articulation problems who received therapy from aides showed changes in articulation scores that were significantly greater than if they had not received therapy.

In a pilot study on the use of communication aides using operant procedures, Engel and Peterson (1970) reported the program had been a success. They reported that the progress made by children in the program was grossly beyond what one would expect due to maturation. The authors reported speech improvement among the experimental group surpassed the progress made by the control group which was being seen by a professional speech clinician.

Technicians were used by Strong (1972) in a portion of the Minnesota Public Schools to perform two tasks usually completed by the speech clinician. The aide's duties consisted of screening school children for speech defects and managing direct therapy with children over eight years old who exhibited frontal or lateral distortion of sibilant phonemes or distortion of the /r/ phoneme. The program included 117 children between the ages of 8 and 18 years. The author reported a high degree of success with the program.

Gallaway (1975) described a three-year project in which paraprofessionals were trained to administer programmed materials to first through fifth grade students who had articulation errors. His findings suggest that paraprofessionals, using preplanned program materials, can enhance the program of the trained professional. The author noted that by using communication aides the clinician has more time to devote to the more difficult speech, hearing and language cases.

From the research reported in the professional literature, it can be shown that the use of communication aides is effective and worthwhile. No doubt there are many variables which can affect the success of programs using technicians, such as: the quality and quantity of training the aide receives, the treatment the aide receives from professionals, the basic type of person the aide is, the age of the aide, and the education and intelligence of the aide. The factors listed above are not the only ones which can and will affect the success of communication aides in a program, but these factors will contribute to the overall stabilization of the effort.

## Summary

It is apparent that the use of communication aides is widespread. Moll (1974) noted that although there are more clinicians available for school programs, the use of supportive personnel is widespread. Technicians are being trained on the job and at institutions of higher education. The main purpose of a communication aide is to provide service in the area of communicative disorders making it possible for the professional to devote more time to the people with complex speech disorders.

Many reported instances of success and satisfaction regarding the use of aides have been reported. However, much more research needs to be completed and information collected in the area of supervision and training of aides. Also, guidelines need to be examined in the area of ethics and standards as the profession continues to grow in its use of communication aides.

Students and supervisors in the clinical setting need to be familiar with the facts surrounding the use of communication aides. Supervisors or other training personnel need to familiarize the student with this area because upon graduation the student may find himself working with and training aides.

Research in this area is still of vital importance if quality supervision of supportive personnel is to be obtained. If supportive personnel are to be used effectively, supervision and training of these aides is a major responsibility of the supervising clinician. It is vital to the success of programs utilizing aides that supervisors also be trained in the supervision of aides. Because the welfare of the client is always a major concern, it is evident that further supervisory requirements need to be established in the area of supervision for communication aides.

## Questions and Issues

1. Explain what a communication aide is and what duties are normally assigned to an aide.

2. In what type of a professional setting would the use of a communication aide be highly desirable? In what type of a professional setting is a communication aide least effective?

3. When communication aides are employed in professional settings, problems may arise. What are the most common types of problems? Discuss how you might prevent these common problems from occurring; and if you could not prevent the problems from occurring, discuss how you would cope with the problems.

4. Some people who have professional degrees in Speech Pathology have served as communication aides. Do you believe a professional person should serve as an aide? Support your position.

5. Write a job description for a communication aide. Be very specific, establish clear limitations and responsibilities for the aide.

# APPENDIX A

# EVALUATION OF CLINICAL SKILLS

University of North Dakota
Speech and Hearing Clinic

EVALUATION OF CLINICAL SKILLS

Student's Name: _____    Supervisor's Name: _____

Date: _____    Number of Clock Hours: _____

Key

| Letter Grade | Terminology | Point Value |
|---|---|---|
| A | Exceptional, Excellent, Superior | 5 |
| B | Very good, Above average | 4 |
| C | Satisfactory, Acceptable, Average | 3 |
| D | Marginal, Weak, Below average | 2 |
| F | Poor, Failing, Not acceptable | 1 |

Evaluation and Diagnostic Skills

|   | 5 | 4 | 3 | 2 | 1 |
|---|---|---|---|---|---|
| 1. Exhibits adequate theoretical background in disorder area(s) . . . . . . . . . . . | | | | | |
| 2. Makes appropriate use of available client background information to plan evaluation procedures . . . . . . . . . . | | | | | |
| 3. Selects and/or designs procedures for a fully inclusive evaluation of client. . . | | | | | |
| 4. Skill in obtaining case history . . . . . . | | | | | |
| 5. Skill in administering evaluation procedures. . . . . . . . . . . . . . . . | | | | | |
| 6. Accuracy of assessment. . . . . . . . . . . | | | | | |
| 7. Modifies evaluation strategy on the basis of client behavior. . . . . . . . . . . . | | | | | |

|   | 5 | 4 | 3 | 2 | 1 |
|---|---|---|---|---|---|

8.  Skill in interpreting results of
    individual tests or procedures . . . . .

9.  Skill in integrating the information
    gathered to determine nature and
    severity of client problem . . . . . . .

10. Skill in generating appropriate
    recommendations and referral
    based on information gathered
    and on the needs of the client . . . . .

11. Skill in counseling parents and/or
    clients. . . . . . . . . . . . . . . . .

Preparation for Therapy

|   | 5 | 4 | 3 | 2 | 1 |
|---|---|---|---|---|---|

1.  Exhibits adequate theoretical background
    in disorder area . . . . . . . . . . . .

2.  Generates appropriate strategies for
    initial contacts on the basis of
    relevant information available . . . . .

3.  Efficiently specifies appropriate direction
    of remedial program on the basis of
    initial contact baseline behavior. . . .

4.  Selects appropriate remedial methodologies
    as an initial framework. . . . . . . . .

5.  Generates appropriate daily goals in a
    logical sequence during planning . . . .

6.  Is aware of, specifies, and controls
    stimulus progression during
    planning . . . . . . . . . . . . . . . .

7.  Is aware of, specifies and controls
    response complexity during
    planning . . . . . . . . . . . . . . . .

8.  Plans for appropriate reinforcement
    (schedule and/or type) . . . . . . . . .

9.  Specifies objective criteria for
    achievement of daily goals . . . . . . .

10. Devises appropriate type and variety
    of materials for the client. . . . . . .

11. Plans for optimum use of materials
    in relation to strategy. . . . . . . . .

Client Management

|   | 5 | 4 | 3 | 2 | 1 |
|---|---|---|---|---|---|
| 1. Efficiently uses therapy time . . . . . . . | | | | | |
| 2. Demonstrates appropriate interaction with the client . . . . . . . . . . . . | | | | | |
| 3. Effectively uses oral language in giving clear and concise directions and information . . . . . . . . . . . . . . . | | | | | |
| 4. Appropriately manipulates stimulus progression during clinical sessions. . . . . . . . . . . . . . . . | | | | | |
| 5. Appropriately manipulates response complexity during clinical sessions. . . . . . . . . . . . . . . . | | | | | |
| 6. Appropriately utilizes reinforcement. . . . | | | | | |
| 7. Client evaluation (accurately monitors and/or records objective information regarding client behavior). . . . . . . . . . . . . | | | | | |
| 8. Makes appropriate recommendations regarding additional client management. . . . . . . | | | | | |

Personal and Professional Qualities

|   | 5 | 4 | 3 | 2 | 1 |
|---|---|---|---|---|---|
| 1. Demonstrates appropriate dress and grooming for professional activity. . . . . . . . . . . . . . . . . | | | | | |
| 2. Is prompt and dependable in meeting professional and practicum responsibilities. . . . . . . . . . . . . | | | | | |
| 3. Demonstrates appropriate writing skills in completing lesson plans, professional and parent contact, reports. . . . . . . . . . . . . . | | | | | |
| 4. Self-evaluation . . . . . . . . . . . . . . | | | | | |
| 5. Interaction with supervisor (seeks supervisory assistance and feedback when appropriate, accepts supervisory assistance, and integrates, adapts, and implements suggestions) . . . . . . . . . | | | | | |

| | 5 | 4 | 3 | 2 | 1 |
|---|---|---|---|---|---|
| 6. Demonstrates appropriate initiative . . . . | | | | | |
| 7. Demonstrates appropriate interaction with parents, other professionals and students. . . . . . . . . . . . . . | | | | | |
| 8. Demonstrates ability and willingness to function independently. . . . . . . . . | | | | | |

COMMENTS:

Grade: _____

_____
(Signature of Student)

_____
(Signature of Supervisor)

# APPENDIX B

# EVALUATION OF SUPERVISION

APPENDIX B

## University of North Dakota
## Speech and Hearing Clinic

### EVALUATION OF SUPERVISION

Supervisor: _____ Date: _____ Semester _____

Key

| Letter Grade | Terminology | Point Value |
|---|---|---|
| A | Exceptional, Excellent, Superior | 5 |
| B | Very good, Above average | 4 |
| C | Satisfactory, Acceptable, Average | 3 |
| D | Marginal, Weak, Below average | 2 |
| F | Poor, Failing, Not acceptable | 1 |

GENERAL COMMENTS

| | 5 | 4 | 3 | 2 | 1 |
|---|---|---|---|---|---|
| 1. Supervisor bases comments objectively . . . . . . . . . . . . . . . | | | | | |
| 2. Supervisor motivates clinician to constructively analyze his/her work and develop independence . . . . . . | | | | | |
| 3. Supervisor relates with clinician and establishes a good working relationship . . . . . . . . . . . . . . | | | | | |
| 4. Supervisor demonstrates understanding of difficult situations, failures, etc. during therapy . . . . . . . . . . . | | | | | |
| 5. Supervisor shows active, personal interest in the clinician's work . . . . . . . . | | | | | |

|   |   |   | 5 | 4 | 3 | 2 | 1 |
|---|---|---|---|---|---|---|---|

6. Supervisor is clear and understandable
   in explanations . . . . . . . . . . . . . . .

7. Supervisor is available for routine
   guidance . . . . . . . . . . . . . . . .

8. Supervisor is available when extra
   help is needed . . . . . . . . . . . . .

9. Supervisor has the ability to deal
   effectively with clinician's
   difficulties and tailors supervision to coincide with level
   of clinician's skill. . . . . . . . . . .

10. Supervisor motivates clinician to do
    her/his best. . . . . . . . . . . . . . .

11. Supervisor is valuable to clinician as a
    teacher of clinical skills. . . . . . . .

LESSON PLANS AND OBSERVATIONS OF THERAPY

|   | Lesson Plans | | | | | Observations | | | | |
|---|---|---|---|---|---|---|---|---|---|---|
|   | 5 | 4 | 3 | 2 | 1 | 5 | 4 | 3 | 2 | 1 |

1. Supervisor understands
   clinician's rationale
   regarding objectives
   and strategies . . . . .

2. Supervisor provides
   verbal feedback on
   therapy objectives
   and strategies and
   alternatives . . . . . .

3. Supervisor provides
   written feedback
   on therapy
   objectives and
   strategies and
   alternatives . . . . . .

4. Supervisor offers
   alternative view-
   points or approaches . .

5. Supervisor offers
   justified explanations
   or rationales for
   comments made. . . . . .

|  | Lesson Plans | | | | | Observations | | | | |
|---|---|---|---|---|---|---|---|---|---|---|
|  | 5 | 4 | 3 | 2 | 1 | 5 | 4 | 3 | 2 | 1 |
| 6. Supervisor provides written feedback on clinician progress during the semester. . . . . . . . . |  |  |  |  |  |  |  |  |  |  |
| 7. Supervisor provides verbal feedback on clinician progress during the semester. . . . . . . . . |  |  |  |  |  |  |  |  |  |  |
| 8. Supervisor encourages clinician freedom to develop own skills and ideas . . . . . . . . . . |  |  |  |  |  |  |  |  |  |  |

Generally, supervision of clinical skills can be viewed as movement from dependence to independence.  The level of supervision then moves from

   Demonstration (show) to
    Verbal or Written Instructions (tell) to
     Asking Questions to Prompt Solutions (consultation) to
      Clinician evaluates (self-supervision)

Which level of supervision would be of most value to you?

Use back for comments.

# BIBLIOGRAPHY

Aiken, L., Relationships of Dress to Selected Measures of Personality in Undergraduate Women. *Journal of Social Psychology*, 59, 119-128 (1963).

Allen, D., and Ryan, K., *Microteaching*. Menlo Park, Calif.: Addison-Wesley Publishing Company, Inc. (1969).

Allen, S.,; Spear, P.; and Lucke, J., Effects of Social Reinforcement on Learning and Retention in Children. *Developmental Psychology*, 5, 73-80 (1971).

Allport, G., and Vernon, P., *Studies in Expressive Behavior*. 2nd Edition. New York: Hafner Publishing Co. (1967).

Alpiner, J.; Ogden, J.; and Wiggins, J., The Utilization of Supportive Personnel in Speech Correction in the Public Schools: A Pilot Project. *Asha*, 12, 599-604 (1970).

Altman, H., A Science Observation System. In Simon, A., and Boyer, E. (Eds.), *Mirrors of Behavior, Vol. VII.* Philadelphia, Penn.: Research for Better Schools (1970).

Ambroe, M., Locating Supervisors for the CFY Experience: A Report for Minnesota. *Asha*, 16, 738 (1974).

American Boards of Examiners in Speech Pathology and Audiology of the American Speech and Hearing Association, *Accreditation of Training Programs Guidelines for Self-Study and Applications.* Washington, D.C.: American Speech and Hearing Association (1969).

American Speech and Hearing Association, Report on Task Force on Supervision. *J. Language, Speech, Hearing Services in the Schools* 3, 4-10 (1972).

Amidon, E., Interaction Analysis. In *Methods of Research in Communication*, ed. by Emmert, P., and Brooks, W. Boston, Mass.: Houghton Mifflin (1970).

Amidon, E., and Flanders, N., *Interaction Analysis: Theory, Research, and Application.* Reading, Mass.: Addison-Wesley (1967).

Amidon, E., and Hough, J., *Interaction Analysis: Theory, Research and Application.* Reading, Mass.: Addison-Wesley Publications (1957).

Amidon, E., and Hunter, E., *Improving Teaching. Analyzing Verbal Interaction in the Classroom.* New York: Holt, Rinehart, and Winston, Inc. (1966).

Amidon, E., and Simon, A., Implications for Teaching Education of Interaction Analysis Research in Student Teaching. Paper presented at the American Educational Research Association Convention, Chicago, Ill. (1965).

Amidon, P., *Nonverbal Interaction Analysis.* Minneapolis, Minn.: P.S. Amidon and Associates (1971).

Anderson, A., An Analysis of Instructor-Student Classroom Interaction. *J. of Med. Ed.*, 41, 209-214 (1966).

Anderson, J., *Handbook for Supervisors of School Practicum in Speech, Hearing and Language.* Bloomington, Ind.: Indiana University (1972a).

———————: Status of Supervision of Speech, Hearing, and Language Programs in the Schools. *Lang., Speech, Hearing Serv. Schools*, 3, 12-22 (1972b).

———————: Status of College and University Programs of Practicum in the Schools. *Asha*, 15, 60-65 (1973).

———————: Supervision: The Neglected Component of Our Profession. In Turton, L. (Ed.), *Proceedings of a Workshop on Supervision in Speech Pathology.* Ann Arbor, Mich.: University of Michigan, Institute for the Study of Mental Retardation and Related Disabilities, Continuing and Adult Education Unit, 4-28 (1973).

———————: Supervision of Schools Speech, Hearing, and Language Programs--An Emerging Role. *Asha*, 16, 7-10 (1974).

———————: *Conference on Supervision of Speech and Hearing Programs in the Schools.* Bloomington, Ind.: Indiana University (1970).

Anderson, J., and Kirtley, D. (Eds.), *Institute on Supervision of Speech and Hearing Programs in the Public Schools.* Indiana: Department of Public Instruction (1966).

Anderson, R.; Struthers, J.; and James, H., Development of a Verbal and Nonverbal Observation Instrument. Paper presented to the American Educational Research Association, Minneapolis, Minn. (1970).

Andrews, J., Applying Principles of Instructional Technology in Evaluating Speech and Language Services. *Lang. Speech Hearing Serv. Schools*, 65-71 (1973).

———————: Operationally Written Therapy Goals in Supervised Clinical Practicum. *Asha*, 13, 385-387 (1971).

Ardey, R., *The Territorial Imperative.* New York: Atheneum House, Inc. (1970).

Argyle, M., *The Psychology of Interpersonal Behavior.* Maryland: Penguin Books (1967).

Argyle, M., and Dean, J., Eye Contact, Distance, and Affiliation. *Sociometry*, 28, 289-304 (1965).

Argyle, M., and Kendon, L., The Experimental Analysis of Social Performance. *Advances in Experimental Social Psych.*, Ed. by Berkowitz, L. New York: Academic Press, 55-98 (1967).

Argyris, C., *Organization and Innovation.* Honeywood, Ill.: Richard D. Irwin, Inc., and The Dorsey Press (1965).

———————: Interpersonal Barriers to Decision Making. *Harvard Bus. Rev.*, 44, 84-97 (1966).

ASHA Committee on Legislation, The Need for Adequately Trained Speech Pathologists and Audiologists. *Asha*, 1, 138-139 (1959).

Aschner, M.; Perry, J.; Jenne, W.; Gallagher, J.; Afsar, S.; and Fau, H. Aschner-Gallagher System. In Simon, A., and Boyer, E. (Eds.), *Mirrors of Behavior, Vol. I.* Philadelphia, Penn.: Research for Better Schools (1967).

Ayer, F., and Pecklam, D., *Check List for Planning and Appraising Supervision.* Austin, Tex.: The Steck Co., Pub. (1948).

Ayres, H., A Baseline Study of Nonverbal Feedback: Observers' Judgments of Audience Members' Attitudes. Doctoral Dissertation, University of Utah, Salt Lake City, Utah (1970).

Backus, O., and Beasley, J., *Speech Therapy with Children*. Boston, Mass.: Houghton Mifflin (1951).

Bailey, K., and Sowder, W., Audiotape and Videotape Self-Confrontation in Psychotherapy. *Psychological Bulletin*, 76, 127-137 (1970).

Bales, R., A Set of Categories for the Analysis of Small Group Interaction. *Am. Soc. Rev.*, 15, 257-263 (1950a).

——————————: *Interaction Process Analysis: A Method for the Study of Small Groups*. Reading, Mass.: Addison-Wesley (1950b).

——————————: *Personality and Interpersonal Behavior*. New York: Holt, Rinehart and Winston (1970).

Bangs, T., and Riser, A., Efficiency in Report Writing. *Hear. Speech News*, 37, 12-16 (1969).

Bankson, N., Report on State Certification Requirements in Speech and Hearing. *Asha*, 10, 291-293 (1968).

Barker, L., and Collins, N., Nonverbal and Kinesic Research. In *Methods of Research in Communication*, Edited by Emmert, P., and Brooks, W. Boston, Mass.: Houghton Mifflin (1970).

Barker, R., and Wright, H., *Recording and Analyzing Child Behavior: With Ecological Data from an American Town*. New York: Harper and Row (1967).

Barnlund, D., Consistency of Emergent Leadership in Groups with Changing Tasks and Members. *Speech Monographs*, 29, 45-52 (1962).

Barnlund, D., and Haiman, F., *The Dynamics of Discussion*. Boston, Mass.: Houghton Mifflin Co. (1960).

Berger, M. (Ed.), *Videotape Techniques in Psychiatric Training and Treatment*. New York: Brunner-Mazel (1970).

Berlo, D., *The Process of Communication*. New York: Holt, Rinehart, and Winston, Inc. (1960).

Berman, L., and Usery, M., *Personalized Supervision: Sources and Insights*. Washington, D.C.: Association for Supervision and Curriculum Development (1966).

Bernstein, L., and Dana, R., *Interviewing and the Health Professions*. New York: Appleton-Century-Crofts (1970).

Bernthal, J., and Beukelman, D., Self-evaluation by the Student Clinician. *The Journal of the National Student Speech and Hearing Association*, 3, 39-44 (1975).

Berry, M., Historical Vignettes of Leaders in Speech and Hearing: I Speech Pathology. *Asha*, 7, 8-9 (1965).

Bietler, R., *Psychology Applied to Teaching*. Boston, Mass.: Houghton Mifflin Company (1974).

Birch, D., Effects of Inquiry Orientation and Guided Self-Analysis Using Videotape on the Verbal Teaching Behavior of Intermediate Grades. Doctoral Dissertation, University of California, Berkeley, Calif. (1969).

Birdwhistell, R., Kinesic Analysis of the Investigation of Emotions. *Expression of the Emotions of Man*, ed. by Knapp, P. New York: International University Press, 123-139 (1963).

————————: *Kinesics and Context; Essays on Body Motion Communication.* Philadelphia, Penn.: University of Pennsylvania Press (1970).

Black, M.; Miller, E.; Anderson, J.; and Coates, N., Supervision of Speech and Hearing Programs. *J. Speech Hearing Dis. Monogr. Suppl.* 8, 32-33 (1961).

Blackburn, H., Effects of Motivating Instructions on Reaction Time in Cerebral Disease. *Journal of Abnormal and Social Psychology,* 56, 359-366 (1958).

Bloom, B.,; Hastings, J.; and Madaus, G.. *Handbook on Formative and Summative Evaluation of Student Learning.* New York: McGraw-Hill (1971).

Bloomer, H., Professional Education in Speech Pathology and Audiology. *Asha,* 10, 255-256 (1968).

————————: Professional Training in Speech Correction and Clinical Audiology. *J. Speech Hearing Dis.,* 21, 5-11 (1956).

Blumberg, A., A System for Analyzing Supervisor-Teacher Interaction. In Simon and Boyer (Eds.), *Mirrors for Behavior: An Anthology of Observation Instruments.* Philadelphia, Penn.: Research for Better Schools, Inc. (1970).

Boone, D., A 'Can Do' Approach to Speech and Language Therapy. *The Journal of the National Student Speech and Hearing Association,* 3, 21-25 (1975).

————————: An Experimental Study of the Acquisition of Behavioral Principles by Videotape Self-Confrontation. Final Report, Project 4071, Grant OEG 8-07139-2814, U.S. Department of Health, Education and Welfare, Division of Research, Bureau of Education for the Handicapped, Office of Education (1969).

Boone, D., and Goldbert, A., An Experimental Study of the Acquisition of Behavioral Principles by Videotape Self-Confrontation. Final Report, Project No. 4071, U.S. Department of Health, Education and Welfare, Division of Research, Bureau of Education for the Handicapped, Office of Education (1969).

Boone, D., and Prescott, T., Application of Videotape and Audiotape Self-Confrontation Procedures to Training Clinicians in Speech and Hearing Therapy, Part II. Denver, Colorado. Final Report of BEH Office of Education Grant OEG-0-70-4758 (1972a).

————————: Content and Sequence Analysis of Speech and Hearing Therapy. *Asha,* 14, 58-62 (1972b).

————————: *Audiotape and Videotape Self-Confrontation Manual.* Denver, Colo.: University of Denver (1970).

————————: *Speech and Hearing Therapy Scoring Manual.* Denver, Colo.: University of Denver (1971).

Boone, D., and Stech, E., *The Development of Clinical Skills in Speech Pathology by Audiotape and Videotape Self-Confrontation.* Denver, Colo.: University of Denver (1970).

Bordeen, J., Interpersonal Perception Through the Tactile, Verbal, and Visual Modes. Paper presented at the International Communication Association Convention, Phoenix, Ariz. (1971).

Brannigan, C., and Humphries, D., Human Non-Verbal Behavior: A Means of Communication. In *Ethological Studies of Infant Behavior.* Edited by Blurton-Jones, N. Cambridge, Mass.: Cambridge University Press (1971).

Brooks, R., and Hannah, E., A Tool for Clinical Supervision. *J. Speech Hearing Dis.*, 31, 383-387 (1966).

Brookshire, R., Speech Pathology and the Experimental Analysis of Behavior. *J. Speech Hearing Dis.*, 32, 215-227 (1967).

Brown, E., Standards for Quality Supervision of Clinical Practicum. In Miner, A. (Ed.), A Symposium: Improving Supervision of Clinical Practicum. *Asha*, 9, 471-481 (1967).

Brown, E.,; Anderson, J.; Dublinski, S.; and Herbert E., ASHA Task Force Report on Supervision in the Schools. *Language Speech Hearing Serv. Schools*, 2, 4-17 (1972).

Brown, E., and Block F., Your Right to Say It. Paper Presented at the American Speech and Hearing Association Convention, Las Vegas, Nev. (1974).

Bryant, D., and Karl, R., *Oral Communication*. New York: Appleton-Century-Crofts (1962).

Buehler, R., and Richmond, J., Interpersonal Communication Behavior Analysis: A Research Method. *Journal of Communication,* 13, 146-155 (1963).

Bugental, D., and Lehner, G., Accuracy of Self-Perception and Group Perception as Related to Two Leadership Roles. *Journal of Abnormal Social Psychology*, 56, 396-398 (1958).

Byrne, M; Shelton, R., Jr.; and Diedrich, W., Articulatory Skill, Physical Management, and Classification of Children with Cleft Palates. *J. Speech Hearing Dis.* 26, 326-333 (1961).

Cairns, R., Informational Properties of Verbal and Nonverbal Events. *Journal of Personality and Social Psychology*, 5, 353-357 (1967).

California Teachers Association, *Six Areas of Teacher Competence*. Burlingame, Calif.: California Teachers Association (1964).

————————: *Teachers Competence: Its Nature and Scope*. Burlingame, Calif.: California Teachers Association (1957).

Caniff, C., and Peiser, K., Rehabilitation Facilities' Needs for Supportive Personnel. *Selection, Training, and Utilization of Supportive Personnel in Rehabilitation Facilities*. Assoc. Rehab. Centers, Evanston, Ill.: 13-20.

Carkhuff, R., *Helping and Human Relations: A Primer for Lay and Professional Helpers. Vol 1. Selection and Training*. New York: Holt, Rinehart and Winston, Inc. (1969a).

————————: *Helping and Human Relations: A Primer for Lay and Professional Helpers. Vol. 2. Practice and Research*. New York: Holt, Rinehart and Winston, Inc. (1969b).

Carnell, C., Criteria for the Evaluation of the Strengths and Weaknesses of Community Speech and Hearing Centers. Paper presented at the American Speech and Hearing Association Convention, Detroit, Mich. (1973).

Carroll, M., An Instrument for Analyzing Activities of Guidance Personnel. *Counselor Educ. Supervision.* 6, 201-204 (1967).

Castle, W., Employment Opportunities in Speech Pathology and Audiology: Fact and Prophecy. *Central States Speech J.*, 27-31 (1967).

Cathcart, R., and Samovar, L., *Small Group Communication: A Reader*. Dubuque, Iowa: Wm. C. Brown Co. (1970).

Caven, C., Supervision: The Supervisee Speaks. Paper presented at the American Speech and Hearing Association Convention, Detroit, Mich. (1973).

Clark, F.; Evans, D.; and Hamerlynch, L., Implementing Behavioral Programs in Schools and Clinics.-*Proceedings of the Third Baniff International Conference on Behavior Modification, Research Press*, Champaign, Ill. (1971).

Clements, R., Art Teacher Student, Questioning and Dialogue in the Classroom. *Classroom Interaction Newsletter*, 2, 22-23 (1967).

Clifford, S., Video Valuable in Speech-Hearing Therapy. *Audecibel*, 17, 168-171 (1967).

Cogan, M., *Clinical Supervision*. Boston, Mass.: Houghton Mifflin Co. (1973).

Colley, K., Psychotherapeutic Process. *Ann. Rev. Psychol.*, 15, 347-370 (1964).

Condon, J., *Semantics and Communication*. London: The Macmillan Company (1969).

Condon, W., and Ogston, W., Sound Film Analysis of Normal and Pathological Behavior Patterns. *Journal of Nervous and Mental Disease*, 143, 338-346 (1966).

Connor, L., Diagnostic Teaching--The Teacher's New Role. *Volta Review*, 61, 311-315 (1959).

Cooper, E., Client-Clinician Relationships and Concomitant Factors in Stuttering Therapy. *J. Speech Hearing Res.*, 9, 194-207 (1966).

Creaner, J., and Gilmore, J., *Design for Competency Based Education in Special Education*. Syracuse, N.Y.: Syracuse University (1974).

Crum, J., and Matkin, N., Room Acoustics: The Forgotten Variable? *Language Speech and Hearing Services in Schools*, 2, 106-110 (1976).

Culatta, R.; Colucci, S.; and Wiggins, E., Clinical Supervisors and Trainees: Two Views of a Process. *Asha*, 17, 152-157 (1975).

Culatta, R., and Seltzer, H., Content and Sequence Analysis of the Supervisory Session. *Asha*, 18= 8-12 (1976).

Curlee, R., Personal Income in the Speech and Hearing Profession. *Asha*, 17, 21-30 (1975).

Curtis, J.; Egan, J.; Hirsh, I.; Matthews, J.; and Peterson, G., Report of Subcommittee on Problems of Basic Research in Speech and Hearing. *J. Speech Hearing Dis., Mono. Supp.* 5, 66-70 (1959).

Dabul, B., Professional Competency and the Student Clinician. *Journal of the National Student Speech and Hearing Association*, 2, 22-26 (1974).

Darley, F., Clinical Training for Full-time Clinical Service: A Neglected Obligation. *Asha*, 11, 142-148 (1969).

——————————: *Diagnosis and Appraisal of Communication Disorders*. Englewood Cliffs, N.J.: Prentice Hall (1964).

——————————: (Ed.), *Graduate Education in Speech Pathology and Audiology*. Washington, D.C.: American Speech and Hearing Association (1963).

——————————: (Ed.), Public School Speech and Hearing Services. *J. Speech Hearing Dis., Monograph Suppl.* 8. Washington, D.C.: American Speech and Hearing Association (1961).

Darley, F., and Moll, K., Reliability of Language Measures and Size of Language Sample. *J. Speech Hearing Res.*, 3, 2, 166-173 (1960).

Darwin, C., *The Expression of Emotion in Man and Animals*. London: Appleton-Century-Crofts (1872).

Davis, G., An Examination of Dialogue and Certain Other Factors and Their Influençe on Interaction Between the Client and the Therapist in the Therapeutic Process in Speech and Hearing. Doctoral Dissertation, Ohio State University, Columbus, Ohio (1968).

Deever, R.; Demeke, H.; and Wochner, R., *The Evaluation of Teaching Competence*. Workshop Manual, IOTA, Fifth Edition. Tempe, Ariz.: Arizona State University (1971).

Diedrich, W., Assessment of the Clinical Process. *J. Kansas Speech Hearing Assoc.*, 10, 1-8 (1969).

———————: Procedures for Counting and Charting a Target Phoneme. *Lang. Speech Hearing Serv. Schools*, 2, 18-32 (1972a).

Diedrich, W., and Crouch, Z., *Programmed Instruction for the Use of Charting in Speech Pathology*. Kansas City, Kansas: University of Kansas (1972b).

———————: Procedures for Counting and Charting a Target Phoneme. In Anderson, J. (Ed.), *Conference on Supervision of Speech and Hearing Programs in the Schools*. Bloomington, Ind.: Indiana University (1970a).

———————: The Use of a Multidimensional Clinical Process Scoring System for Training Students in Speech Pathology. Paper presented at meeting, Videotape and Audiotape Confrontation in Clinical Training. University of Denver, Denver, Colo. (1970b).

———————: Use of Videotape in Teaching Clinical Skills. *Volta Rev.*, 644-647 (1966).

Dierssen, G.; Lorenc, M.; and Spitalerl, R., A New Method for Graphic Study of Human Movements. *Neurology*, 2, 610-618 (1961).

DiSimoni, F., A Proposed Model for Evaluating Clinician Performance. *Journal of the Minn. Speech and Hearing Assoc.*, 3, 12, 117-125 (1975).

Dittman, A., and Llewellyn, L., Relationship Between Vocalization and Head Nods as Listener Response. *Journal of Personality and Social Psychology*, 9, 79-84 (1968).

Duncan, S., Nonverbal Communication. *Psychological Bulletin*, 72, 118-137 (1969).

Dussault, J., *A Theory of Supervision in Teacher Education*. New York: Teachers College, Columbia University (1970).

Eagly, A., Leadership Style and Role Differentiation as Determinates of Group Effectiveness. *Journal of Personality*, 38, 509-524 (1970).

Egolf, B., and Chester, S., Nonverbal Communication and the Disorders of Speech and Language. *Asha*, 15, 511-518 (1973).

Eisenberg, S., and Delaney, D., Using Video Stimulation of Counseling for Trained Counselors. *Journal of Consulting Psychology*, 17, 15-19 (1970).

Eisenstadt, A., Weakness in Clinical Procedures--A Parental Evaluation. *Asha*, 14, 7-9 (1972).

Ekman, P., Communication Through Nonverbal Behavior: A Source of Information About an Interpersonal Relationship. *Affect, Cognition and Personality*. Edited by Tomkins, S., and Igard, C. New York: Springer (1965).

———————: A Methodological Discussion of Nonverbal Behavior. *Journal of Psychology*, 53, 141-149 (1957).

Ekman, P., and Friesen. W., A Tool for the Analysis of Motion Picture Film or Video Tape. *American Psychologist*, 24, 240-243 (1969a).
————————: The Repertoire of Nonverbal Behavior: Categories, Origins, Usage, and Coding. *Semiotica*, 1, 49-98 (1969b).
Ekman, P.; Friesen, W., and Taussign, T., VIO-R and SCAN: Tools and Methods in the Analysis of Facial Expression and Body Movement. In *Content Analysis*, Edited by Gerbner, G.; Holst, O.; Krippendorf, K.; Paisley, W.; and Stone, P. New York: Wiley (1969).
Ekman, P.; Friesen, W.; and Tomkins, S., Facial Affect Scoring Technique: A First Validity Study. *Semiotica*, 3, 37-58 (1971).
Elliott, L., and Vergely, A., Notes on Clinical Record-Keeping System. *Asha*, 8, 444-446 (1971).
Ellsworth, P., and Ledwig, L., Visual Behavior in Social Interaction. *Journal of Communication*, 22, 375-403 (1972).
Emerick, L., *The Parent Interview, Guidelines for Students and Practicing Speech Clinicians*. Danville, Ill.: Interstate (1969).
Emerick, L., and Hatten, J., *Diagnosis and Evaluation in Speech Pathology*, Englewood Cliffs, N.J.: Prentice-Hall (1974).
Engel, D., and Peterson, D., A Pilot Study Using a Teacher Aide Employing Operant Procedures to Assist a Speech Clinician in a Public School Setting. *Teacher and His Staff*, 102-106 (1970).
————————: The Use of An Operant Procedure by a Teacher Aide in a Public School Setting. Paper presented at the American Speech and Hearing Association Convention, Chicago, Ill. (1969).
English, R., and Lillywhite, H., A Semantic Approach to Clinical Reporting in Speech Pathology. *Asha*, 5, 647-650 (1963).
Engnoth, J., and Lingwall, J., A Comparison of Three Approaches to Supervision of Speech Clinicians. Paper presented at the American Speech and Hearing Association Convention, San Francisco, Calif. (1972).
Erickson, R., and Van Riper, D., Demonstration Therapy in a University Training Program. *Asha*, 9, 33-35 (1961).
Exline, R., Explorations in the Process of Person Perception: Visual Interaction in Relation to Competition, Sex, and Need for Affiliation. *Journal of Personality*, 31, 1-20 (1963).
Exline, R.; Gray, D.; and Schuette, D., Visual Behavior in a Dyad as Affected by Interview Content and Sex of Respondent. *Journal of Personality and Social Psychology*. 1, 201-209 (1965).
Eye, G.; Netzer, L.; and Krey, R., *Supervision of Instruction*. (2nd ed.) New York: Harper and Rowe (1971).
Fabun, D., *Communications: The Transfer of Meaning*. Beverly Hills, Calif.: The Glencoe Press (1968).
Falck, V., The Roll and Function of University Training Programs. *Asha*, 14, 307-310 (1972).
Fankhouser, C., and Katsarkas, A., Employment of Technicians in Diagnostic Audiometry. *Hearing and Speech Action*, 44, 20-23 (1976).
Fast, J., *Body Language*. New York: M. Evans & Co., Inc. (1970).
Faules, D., The Relation of Communicator Skill to the Ability to Elicit and Interpret Feedback Under Four Conditions. *Journal of Communication*, 17, 362-371 (1967).

Fisher, L., Reporting: In the School to the Community. In Van Hattum, R. (Ed.), *Clinical Speech in the Schools*. Springfield, Ill.: Charles C. Thomas (1969).

Flanders, N., *Analyzing Teaching Behavior*. Reading, Mass.: Addison-Wesley Pub. Co. (1970).

——————: *Classroom Interaction Patterns, Pupil Attitudes, and Achievement in the Second, Fourth and Sixth Grades*. Cooperative Research Project No. 5-1055 (OE 4-10-243), U.S. Office of Ed., Ann Arbor, Mich.: The University of Michigan, School of Ed. (1969).

——————: *Helping Teachers Change Their Behavior*. Final Report, NDEA Projects 1721012 and 7-32-0560-171.0, U.S. Office of Ed., Ann Arbor, Mich.: The University of Michigan, School of Ed. (1963).

——————: *Teacher Influence in the Classroom*. In Amidon, E., and Hough, J. (Eds.), *Interaction Analysis: Theory, Research, and Application*. Reading, Mass.: Addison-Wesley Pub. Co. (1967).

Flower, R. (Ed.), *Conference on Standards for Supervised Experience for Speech and Hearing Specialists in Public Schools*. Orange County, Department of Education, Los Angeles, Calif. (1969).

Forsdale, L., *Nonverbal Communication*. New York: Harcourt Brace Jovanovich, Inc. (1974).

Fowler, H., *Modern English Usage*. London: Oxford University Press (1957).

Frahm, J., Verbal-Nonverbal Interaction Analysis: Exploring a New Methodology for Quantifying Dyadic Communication Systems. Doctoral Dissertation, Michigan State University, East Lansing, Mich. (1970).

Frank, L., Tactile Communication. *Genetic Psychology Monograph*, 56, 209-255 (1957).

Frederick-Middleton, G., and Pannbacker, M., Supervision—A Paradox. Paper presented at the American Speech and Hearing Association Convention, Washington, D.C. (1973).

Freed, H., On Various Uses of the Recorded Interview in Psychotherapy. *Psychiat. Quart.*, 22, 685-695 (1948).

Freidrick, G., and Brooks, W., The Use of Systemic Observational Instrument for the Supervision of Teachers. *Speech Teacher*, 18, 283 (1970).

Fricke, J.; Johnson, K.; and Castle, W., Personal Incomes in the Speech and Hearing Profession: Academic Faculty. *Asha*, 11, 44-50 (1969).

Fricke, J.; Johnson, K.; and Tiffany, W., The Status of Education and Training Programs in Speech Pathology and Audiology--1968-1969. *Asha*, 12, 287-291 (1970).

Fuller, F., *FAIR System Manual: Fuller Affective Interaction Records*. Austin, Tex.: University of Texas, Research and Development Center for Teacher Evaluation (1969).

Gallaway, F., Jr., and Blue, M., Paraprofessional Personnel in Articulation Therapy. *LSHSS*, 6, 125-130 (1975).

Gardiner, J., A Synthesis of Experimental Studies of Speech Communication Feedback. *Journal of Communication*, 21, 17-35 (1971).

Gardner, J., *Excellence*. New York: Harper and Row (1961).

Gendlin, E., and Rychalk, J., Psychotherapeutic Process. *Annual Review of Psychology*, 21, 156 (1970).

Geocaris, K., The Patient as a Listener. *Arch. Gen. Psychiat.*, 2, 81-88 (1960).

Geoffrey, V., *Report on Supervisory Practices in Speech and Hearing.* College Park, Md.: University of Maryland (1973).

Gewirtz, J., and Baer, D., The Effect of Brief Social Deprivation on Behaviors for a Social Reinforcer. *Journal of Abnormal Social Psychology,* 56, 49-56 (1958a).

Giles, A., The Use of Interaction Analysis in the Training of Speech Therapists. Paper presented at the American Speech and Hearing Association Convention, Chicago, Ill. (1971).

Glanzer, M., and Glanzer, R., Techniques for the Study of Group Structure and Behavior: Empirical Studies of the Effects of Structure in Small Groups. *Psychology Bulletin,* 58, 1-27 (1967).

Glasser, W., *Schools Without Failure.* New York: Harper and Row (1969).

Glick, A., Videotape: An Effective Tool in Speech Pathology. *The North Dakota Speech and Hearing Journal,* 15, 5-18 (1972).

Goldberg, S., The Development of Competency-Based Training Programs in Speech Pathology. Paper presented at the American Speech and Hearing Association Convention, Las Vegas, New. (1974).

Goldhammer, R., *Clinical Supervision.* New York: Holt, Rinehart, and Winston, Inc. (1969).

Good, R., The Written Language of Rehabilitation Medicine: Meanings and Usages. *Archs. Phys. Med. Rehabil.,* 51, 29-36 (1970).

Gordon, K.; Cooper, T.; and Williams, G., A Precision Therapy Skillshop: A Competency Based In-Service Instructional Module for Speech Clinicians and Supervisors. Paper presented at the American Speech and Hearing Association Convention, Detroit, Mich. (1973).

Graves, H., and Hoffman, L., *Report Writing.* Englewood Cliffs, N.J.: Prentice-Hall, 4th ed. (1965).

Greene, L., *Supervision of the Special Subjects.* Milwaukee, Wisc.: The Brue Publishing Company (1922).

Greene, M., Speech Therapy in the British Isles. *Brit. J. of Dis. of Comm.,* 180-185 (1970).

Griffith, F., Philosophy of Clinical Practicum. PHS Training Grant N505362, National Institute of Neurological Disease and Stroke, Bureau of Child Research, University of Kansas, Lawrence, Kansas (1970).

Grossman, P., and Kruse, R., Communication Processes in Clinical Supervision. Paper presented at the American Speech and Hearing Association Convention, Las Vegas, Nev. (1974).

Guion, R., Open a New Window: Validities and Values in Psychological Measurement. *Amer. Psychol.,* 29, 287-296 (1974).

Gulley, H., *Discussion, Conference, and Group Process.* New York: Holt, Rinehart and Winston, Inc. (1968).

Gwynn, J., *Theory and Practice of Supervision.* New York: Dodd, Mead and Company (1961).

Hagen, C.; Porter, W.; and Brink, J., Nonverbal Communication: An Alternate Mode of Communication for the Child with Severe Cerebral Palsy. *Journal of Speech and Hearing Disorders,* 38, 449-455 (1973).

Haggard, E., and Isaacs, K., Micromomentary Facial Expression as Indicators of Ego Mechanisms in Psychotherapy. In *Methods of Research in Psychotherapy,* edited by Gothschalk, A., and Auerback, A. New York: Appleton-Century-Crofts (1966).

Hahn, E., Communication in the Therapy Session: A Point of View. *Journal of Speech and Hearing Disorders*, 25, 18-23 (1960).
——————: Indications for Direct, Non-Direct and Indirect Methods in Speech Correction. *Journal of Speech and Hearing Disorders*, 26, 230-236 (1961).

Haiman, F., The Specialization of Roles and Functions in a Group. *Quarterly Journal of Speech*, 43, 165-173 (1957).

Halfond, M., Clinical Supervision--Stepchild in Training. *Asha*, 6, 441-444 (1964).

Hall, A., The Effectiveness of Videotape Recordings as an Adjunct to Supervision of Clinical Practicum by Speech Pathologists. Doctoral Dissertation, Ohio State University, Columbus, Ohio (1970).

Hall, E., A System for the Notation of Proxemic Behavior. *American Anthropologist*, 65, 1003-1026 (1963).

Haller, R., Standards for Quality Supervision of Clinical Practicum. In Miner, A. (Ed.), A Symposium: Improving Supervision of Clinical Practicum. *Asha*, 9, 471-481 (1967).

Ham, R. (Ed.), *The Ohio Project on Supportive Personnel in Speech Pathology and Audiology*. Athens, Ohio: School of Speech and Hearing Sciences, Ohio University, Athens, Ohio (1968).

Hammond, K., and Allen, J., *Writing Clinical Reports*. Englewood Cliffs, N.J.: Prentice-Hall (1953).

Hamre, C., Research and Clinical Practice: A Unifying Model. *Asha*, 14, 542-545 (1972).

Hardy, J., and Counihan, D., The Certificate of Clinical Competence: A Status Report and Suggestions for Obtaining It. *Asha*, 13, 601-606 (1971).

Hare, E.; Borgatte, F.; and Bales, R., *Small Group Studies in Social Interaction*. New York: Appleton-Century-Crofts (1964).

Harrison, R., Verbal-Nonverbal Interaction Analysis: The Substructure of an Interview. Paper presented at the Association for Education in Journalism, Berkeley, Calif. (1969)

Hatfield, M., Supervision: The Supervisee Speaks. Paper presented at the American Speech and Hearing Association Convention, Detroit, Mich. (1973).

Hatfield, M.; Bartlett, C.; Caven, C.; and Veberle, J., Supervision: The superviser Speaks. Paper presented at the American Speech and Hearing Association Convention, Detroit, Mich. (1973).

Hayakawa, S., *Language in Thought and Action*. New York: Harcourt Brace Jovanovich, Inc. (1964).

Haynes, W., and Hartman, D., The Agony of Report Writing: A New Look at an Old Problem. *The Journal of the National Student Speech and Hearing Association*, 3, 7-15 (1975).

Herbert, E., Hearing Impared Children in Community Recreation and Camping Programs. *J. Speech Hearing Dis.*, 23, 610-614 (1958).

Herbert, J., *A System for Analyzing Lessons*. New York: Teachers College Press, Columbia University (1967).

Hersey, P., and Blanchard, K., *Management of Organizational Behavior: Utilizing Human Resources*. Englewood Cliffs, N.J.: Prentice-Hall, Inc. (1969).

Higgins, W.; Ivey, A.; and Uhlemann, M., Media Therapy, A Programmed Approach to Teaching Behavioral Skills. *Journal of Counseling Psychology*, 17, 20-26 (1970).

Hilgard, E., and Bower, J., *Theories of Learning*. New York: Meredith (1966).

Hill, W., *HIM: Hill Interaction Matrix*. Los Angeles, Calif.: Youth Studies Center, University of Southern California (1965).

Hoffman, B., *The Tyranny of Testing*. New York: Crowell-Collier (1962).

Holland, A., Some Application of Behavioral Principles to Clinical Speech Problems. *J. Speech Hearing Dis.*, 32, 11-18 (1967).

Holland, J., and Richards, J., Academic and Nonacademic Accomplishment and Correlated or Uncorrelated? *Journal of Educational Psychology*, 56, 165-174 (1965).

Holt, J., *How Children Fail*. New York: Pittman (1964).

Holzman, P., On Hearing and Seeing Onself. *J. Nerv. Ment. Dis.*, 148, 198-209 (1969).

Holzman, P.; Berger, A.; and Rousey, C., Voice Confrontation: A Bilingual Study. *J. Personality Soc. Psychol.*, 7, 423-428 (1967).

Holzman, P., and Rousey, C., The Voice as a Percept. *J. Personality Soc. Psychol.*, 4, 79-86 (1966).

Holzman, P.: Rousey, C.; and Synder, C., On Listening to One's Own Voice: Effects on Psychophysiological Responses and Free Associations. *J. Personality Soc. Psychol.*, 4, 432-441 (1966).

Honigman, F., and Stevens, J., *Analyzing Student Functioning in an Individualized Instructional Setting*. Final Report: Demonstration Project in the Process of Educating Adult Migrants, Fort Lauderdale, Fla.: Nea Rad, Inc. (1969).

Horowitz, F., Social Reinforcement Effects of Child Behavior. *Journal of Nursery Education*, 18, 276-284 (1963).

Hough, J., An Observational System for the Analysis of Classroom Instruction and Classroom Interaction and the Facilitation of Learning: The Source of Instruction Theory. In Amidon, E., and Hough, J. (Eds.), *Interaction Analysis: Theory, Research, and Application*. Reading, Mass.: Addison-Wesley Pub. Co. (1967).

Huber, J., *Report Writing in Psychology and Psychiatry*. New York: Harper (1961).

Ingmire, S., and Schuckers, G., The Category and Frequency of Verbal Reinforcement Utilized by Clinicians in Schools. Paper presented at the American Speech and Hearing Association Convention, Washington, D.C. (1975).

Ingram, D., and Studen, A., Student's Attitudes Toward the Therapeutic Process. *Asha*, 9, 435-442 (1967).

Irwin, J., Speech Pathology and Behavior Modification. *Acta Symbolica*, 1, 15-23 (1970).

———————————: Supportive Personnel in Speech Pathology and Audiology. *Asha*, 9, 348=354 (1967).

Irwin, R., Behaviors of Speech Clinicians During the Clinical Process. Paper presented at the American Speech and Hearing Association Convention, Washington, D.C. (1975).

———————————: Interactional Analysis of Verbal Behaviors of Supervisors and Speech Clinicians During Microcounseling Sessions. Paper presented at the American Speech and Hearing Association Convention, Detroit, Mich. (1973).

————————: Microsupervision: A Study of the Behaviors of Supervisors of Speech Clinicians. Paper presented at the American Speech and Hearing Association Convention, Chicago, Ill. (1971).

Irwin, R., and Hall, A., Behavior of Speech Clinicians. Paper presented at the American Speech and Hearing Association Convention, San Francisco, Calif. (1972).

Irwin, R., and Nickles, A., The Use of Audiovisual Films in Supervised Observation. *Asha*, 12, 363-367 (1970).

Irwin, R.; Van Riper, C.; Breakey, M.; and Fitzsimons, R., Professional Standards and Training. *J. Speech Hearing Dis., Mono. Supp.* 8, 93-104 (1961).

Isaac, S., and Michael, W., *Handbook in Research and Evaluation*. San Diego, Calif.: Knapp (1972).

Ivey, A; Normington, C.; Miller, C.; Morrill, W.; and Haase, R., Microcounseling and Attending Behavior: An Approach to Prepracticum Counselor Training. *Journal of Counseling Psychology*, 15, 1-12 (1968).

James, W., A Study of the Expression of Bodily Posture. *Journal of General Psychology*, 7, 405-437 (1932).

Jantzen, J., and Stone, J., More Effective Supervision of Beginning Teachers. *J. Teacher Ed.*, 246-248 (1959).

Jason, H., A Study of Medical Teaching Practices. *J. of Med. Ed.*, 37, 1258-1284 (1962).

Jerger, J., Scientific Writing Can Be Readable. *Asha*, 4, 101-104 (1962).

Johnson, K. (Ed.), Requirements for the Certificate of Clinical Competence. *Asha*, 15, 77-90 (1973).

Johnson, T., The Development of a Multidimensional Scoring System for Observing in the Clinical Process in Speech Pathology. In Johnson, T. (Ed.), *Clinical Interaction and Its Measurement*. Logan, Utah: Department of Communicative Disorders, Utah State University (1971).

Johnson, W.; Darley, F.; and Spriestersbach, D., *Diagnostic Methods in Speech Pathology*. New York: Harper and Row (1961).

Johnson, M., and Harris, F., Observation and Recording of Verbal Behavior in Remedial Speech Work. In Sloane, H., and MacAulay, B. (Eds.), *Operant Procedures In Remedial Speech and Language Training*. New York: Houghton Mifflin (1968).

Jones F., and Hanson J., Time-Space Pattern in a Gross Body Movement. *Perceptual and Motor Skills*, 12, 35-41 (1961).

Jones, F., and Nara, M., Interrupted Light Photography to Record The Effect of Changes in the Poise of the Head Upon Patterns of Movement and Posture in Man. *Journal of Psychology*, 40, 125-131 (1955).

Jones, F.; O'Connell, D.; and Hanson, J., Color-Coded Multiple Image Photography for Studying Related Rates of Movement. *Journal of Psychology*, 45, 247-251 (1958).

Jones, E., *Writing Scientific Papers and Reports*. Dubuque, Iowa: Wm. C. Brown Co., 6th Ed (1971).

Jourard, S., An Exploratory Study of Body Accessibility. *British Journal of Social and Clinical Psychology*, 5, 221-231 (1966).

Journot, V., *The Tabulated Accountability Plan for Speech Therapy Services*. Hurst, Tex.: Tabulated Accountability Plan (1973).

Kadushin, A., Games People Play in Supervison. *Social Work*, 3, 23-33 (1968).

Kagan, N., Can Technology Help Us Toward Reliability in Influencing Human Interaction? *Educational Technology*, 44-45 (1973).

——————————: Human Relationships in Supervision. *Conference on Supervision of Speech and Hearing Programs in the Schools*. Bloomington, Ind.: Indiana University (1970).

Kanfer, F., and Karas C., Prior Experimenter-Subject Interaction and Verbal Conditioning. *Psychological Reports*, 5, 345-353 (1959).

Kanfer, I., and Saslow, G., Behavior Analysis: An Alternative to Diagnostic Classification. *Archives of General Psychiatry*, 12, 529-538 (1965).

Kaplan, N., and Dryer, D., The Training of Interpersonal Skill Acquisition in Student Therapists. Paper presented at the American Speech and Hearing Association Convention, Chicago, Ill. (1971).

Kelly, C., Listening: Complex of Activities--and a Unitary Skill? *Speech Monographs*, 34 464 (1967).

Kendon, A., Progress Report of an Investigation into Aspects of the Structure and Function of the Social Performance in Two-Person Encounters. Cited in Argyle, M., *Social Interaction*. New York: Atherton (1969).

King, R., Supervision at a University Training Center. *Speech Teach*. 14, 178-180 (1965).

King, R., and Berger, K., in Ch. 4, Student Conference, 103-110, *Diagnostic Assessment and Counseling Techniques for Speech Pathologists and Audiologists*. Pittsburgh, Penn.: Stanwix (1971).

Kinsinger, R., Education and Training for Technicians in the Health Field. *Selection, Training, And Utilization of Supportive Personnel in Rehabilitation Facilities*. Assoc. Rehab. Centers, Evanston, Ill.: 3-12.

Kirk, R., Experimental Design. *Procedures for the Behavioral Sciences*. Belmont, Calif.: Brooks/Cole Publishing Co. (1968).

Kirtley, D. (Ed.), *Supervision of Student Teaching in Speech and Hearing Therapy*. Indianapolis, Ind.: Department of Public Instruction (1967).

Kleffner, F. (Ed.), *Seminar on Guidelines for the Internship Year*. Washington, D.C.: American Speech and Hearing Association (1964).

Klevens, D., and Volz, H., Development of a Clinical Evaluation Procedure. *Asha*, 16, 489-491 (1974).

Klinkhamer, G., Nonprofessionals in Special Education. Paper presented at the American Speech and Hearing Association Convention, Washington, D.C.: (1966).

Knapp, M., *Nonverbal Communication in Human Interaction*. New York: Holt, Rinehart, and Winston, Inc. (1972).

Knepflar, K., Is Full-Time Private Practice for You? *California Journal of Communicative Disorders*, 2, 143-146 (1972).

——————————: *Report Writing in the Field of Communication Disorders: A Handbook for Students and Clinicians*. Danville, Ill.: The Interstate Printers and Publishers, Inc. (1976).

Knight, H., Function of the School Clinician. *Lang. Speech Hearing Serv. Schools*, 1, 12-17, 20-23 (1970).

Knutson, T., An Experimental Study of the Effects of Orientation Behaviors on Small Group Consensus. *Speech Monographs*, 39, 159-165 (1972).

Krasner, L., Studies on the Conditioning of Verbal Behavior. *Psychological Bulletin*, 55, 148-168 (1958).

Krout, M., An Experimental Attempt to Produce Unconscious Manual Symbolic Movements. *Journal of General Psychology*, 51, 121-152 (1954).

Kunze, L., Standards for Quality Supervision of Clinical Practicum. In Miner, A. (Ed.), A Symposium: Improving Supervision of Clinical Practicum. *Asha*, 9, 471-481 (1967).

Laguaite, J.; Riviere, M.; and Fuller, C., Problems of Terminology. *Asha*, 7, 152-155 (1965).

Larson, C., Forms of Analysis and Small Group Problem-Solving. *Speech Monographs*, 37, 452-455 (1969).

——————————: The Speech Communication Research on Small Groups. *Speech Teacher*, 20, 89 (1971).

Lee, I., *How To Talk With People*. New York: Harper and Row Publishers (1952).

——————————: *Language Habits in Human Affairs*. New York: Harper and Row Publishers (1941).

——————————: *The Language of Wisdom and Folly*. San Francisco, Calif.: International Society for General Semantics (1967).

Leeper, R., Editor, *Educational Leadership, Journal of the Association for Supervision and Curriculum Development*. Washington, D.C.: Association for Supervision and Curriculum Development, NEA, 1201 Sixteenth Street, N.W. (1966).

Leith, W., Clinical Training in Stuttering Therapy: A Survey. *Asha*, 13, 6-8 (1971).

Lewis, M.; Well, M.; and Aronfreed, J., Developmental Change in The Relative Values of Social and Nonsocial Reinforcement. *Journal of Experimental Psychology*, 66, 133-137 (1963).

Lindvall, C.; Yeager, J.; Wang, M.; and Wood, C., Manual for Individually Prescribed Instruction Student Observation Form. In Simon, A., and Boyer, E. (Eds.), *Mirrors of Behavior*, Vol. III. Philadelphia, Penn.: Research for Better Schools (1967).

Lofland, J., *Analyzing Social Settings*. Belmont, Calif.: Wadsworth (1971).

Longabaugh, R., *Resource Process Coding 1969: Its Relevance to the Classroom*. Belmont, Mass.: McLean Hospital (1969).

MacDonald, W., *Battle in the Classroom*. Scranton, Penn.: Intext Educational Publications (1971).

Mackie, R., and Johnson, W. (Eds.), *Speech Correctionists: The Competencies They Need for the Work They Do*. Office of Education Bulletin No. 19, 1-77 (1957).

MacLeanie, E., Appraisal Form for Speech and Hearing Therapists. *J. Speech Hearing Dis.*, 23, 612-614 (1958).

Mager, R., *Goal Analysis*. Belmont, Calif.: Fearon Press (1972).

——————————: *Preparing Instructional Objectives*. Palo Alto, Calif.: Fearon Publishers, Inc. (1962).

Maier, N., *Problem Solving Discussions and Conferences*. New York: McGraw-Hill Book Co. (1963).

Manyuk, P.; Tikofsky, R.; Winitz, H.; and Garrett, E., Speech Pathology: Some Principles Underlying Therapeutic Practices (Report from the American Association for the Advancement of Science Meeting. *Asha*, 10, 200-206 (1968).

Markle, S., *Good Frames and Bad: A Grammar of Frame Writing*. New York: Wiley (1964).

Marshall, N., and Hegrenes, J., The Application of Videotape Replay in Academic and Clinic Settings. *Ment. Retard.*, 8, 17-19 (1970).

Martin, E., Client Centered Therapy as a Theoretical Orientation for Speech Therapy. *Asha*, 5, 576-578 (1963).

Matarazzo, J., Prescribed Behavior Therapy: Suggestions from Interview Research. In Backrach, A., (Ed.), *Experimental Foundation of Clinical Psychology*, New York: Basic Books, 471-509 (1962).

Matthews, J., Essentials of an Acceptable Program of Training for Speech Pathologists and Audiologists. *Asha*, 8, 231-234 (1966).

McCroskey, J., and Wright, D., The Development of an Instrument for Measuring Interaction Behavior in Small Groups. *Speech Monographs*, 38, 335-340 (1971).

McReynolds, L., Reinforcement Procedures for Establishing and Maintaining Echoic Speech by a Non-Verbal Child. In Girardeau, F., and Spradlin, J. (Eds.), *The Functional Analysis Approach to Speech and Language*. Asha Monograph, 14, 60-66 (1970).

Mehrabian, A., Inference of Attitudes from the Posture, Orientation, and Distance of a Communicator. *Journal of Counsulting and Clinical Psychology*, 32, 296-308 (1968a).

———————————: Communication with Words. *Psychology Today*, 52-55 (1968b).

———————————: Methods and Designs: Some Referents and Measures of Nonverbal Behavior. *Behavioral Research Methodology and Instrumentation*, 1, 203-207 (1969).

———————————: A Semantic Space for Nonverbal Behavior. *Journal of Consulting and Clinical Psychology*, 35, 248-257 (1970).

———————————: *Silent Messages*. Belmont, Calif.: Wadsworth Publishing Company, Inc. (1971).

Mehrabian, A., and Williams, M., Nonverbal Concomitants of Perceived and Intended Persuasiveness. *Journal of Personality and Social Psychology*, 13, 37-58 (1969).

Melbin, M., Field Method and Techniques: An Interaction Recording Device for Participant Observers. *Human Organ.*, 13, 29-33 (1954).

Mercer, A., and Schubert, G., Nonverbal Behaviors of Speech Pathologists in the Therapy Setting. Paper distributed at the International Communication Association Convention, New Orleans, La. (1974).

Merrill, P., The Principles of Poor Writing. *Scientific Monthly*, 64, 72-74 (1947).

Michalak, D., The Supervisory Conference on Student Teaching. *Supervisor's Quarterly*, 31-34 (1969).

Milner, E., *The Supervising Teacher*. Dubuque, Iowa: Wm. C. Brown Co., Inc. (1959).

Miner, A., Standards for Quality Supervision of Clinical Practicum. In Miner, A. (Ed.), A Symposium: Improving Supervision of Clinical Practicum. *Asha*, 9, 471-481 (1967).

Minor, G., *Theory and Practice of Supervision*. New York: Dodd Mean and Co. (1961).

Minteer, C., *Words and What They Do To You*. Lakeville, Conn.: Institute of General Semantics (1965).

Moll, K., Issues Facing Us--Supportive Personnel. *Asha,* 16, 358-359 (1974).

Moncur, J., Guidelines on the Role, Training, and Supervision of The Communication Aide. *Asha,* 12, 78-80 (1970).

——————: (Ed.) *Institute on the Utilization of Supportive Personnel in School Speech and Hearing Programs.* Washington, D.C.: American Speech and Hearing Association (1967).

Moore, M., Pathological Writing. *Asha,* 11, 535-538 (1969).

Morris, D., *The Human Zoo.* New York: McGraw-Hill Book Co. (1969).

Mosher, R., and Purpel, D., *Supervision: The Reluctant Profession.* Boston, Mass.: Houghton Mifflin Co. (1972).

Moskowitz, G., The Flint System (Foreign Language Interaction System): An Observational Tool for the Foreign Language Class. In Simon, A., and Boyer, E. (Eds.), *Mirrors of Behavior,* Vol. IV. Philadelphia, Penn,: Research for Better Schools (1967).

Moustakas, G.; Sigel, I.; and Schalock, H., An Analysis of Therapist-Child Interaction in Play Therapy. *Child Dev.,* 22, 143-157 (1955).

Mowrer, D., Accountability and Speech Therapy in the Public Schools. *Asha,* 14, 111-115 (1972).

——————: A Behavorists Approach to Modification of Articulation. In Wolfe, W., and Goulding, D. (Eds.), *Articulation and Learning.* Springfield, Ill.: Charles C. Thomas (1973a).

——————: An Analysis of Motivational Techniques Used in Speech Therapy. *Asha,* 12, 491-493 (1973b).

——————: *Developing Precision in Recording Speech Behaviors.* Salt Lake City, Utah: Word Making Productions (1971).

——————: Evaluating Speech Therapy Through Precision Recording. *J. Speech Hearing Dis.,* 34, 239-244 (1969).

——————: Verbal Content Analysis of Speech Therapy Sessions. Paper presented at the American Speech and Hearing Association Convention, Denver, Colo. (1968).

Mowrer, D.; Baker, R.; and Owen, C., Verbal Content Analysis of Speech Therapy Sessions. Paper presented at the American Speech and Hearing Association Convention, Denver, Colo. (1968).

Mueller, P., and Peters, T., A Clinical Record-Keeping System. *Asha,* 18, 352-353 (1976).

Mulhern, S., and Friedman, P., Relationship of Clinical Reinforcement to Spontaneous Child Verbalization During Language Training. Paper presented at the American Speech and Hearing Association Convention, San Francisco, Calif. (1972).

National IOTA Council, *The Role of the Teacher in Society.* Tempe, Ariz.: Arizona State University (1970).

Naylor, R., Certification and Clinical Practicum (Letter to the Editor). *Asha,* 4, 146 (1964).

Nelson, G., Does Supervision Make a Difference? Paper presented at the American Speech and Hearing Association Convention, Las Vegas, Nev. (1974).

——————: Supervised Training in Clinical Supervision. Paper presented at the American Speech and Hearing Association Convention, San Francisco, Calif. (1972).

————————: University Supervision of Clinical Practicum in Speech and Language Pathology: Let's Set Some Standards! Paper presented at the American Speech and Hearing Association Convention, Detroit, Mich. (1973).

Nickles, A., Judging Clinician Behavior in Speech Pathology. Unpublished Doctoral Dissertation, Denver University, Denver, Colo. (1970).

Nierenberg, G., *The Art of Negotiating.* New York: Hawthorn Books, Inc. (1968).

Nierenberg, G., and Calero, H., *How to Read a Person Like a Book.* New York: Hawthorn Books, Inc. (1971).

Nuttall, E., When Should Clinical Practice Begin? *Asha,* 6, 207-208 (1964).

Oliver, D., and Shaver, J., *The Analysis of Public Controversy: A Study in Citizenship Education.* Cambridge, Mass.: Harvard Graduate School of Ed. (1962).

Olsen, B., Comparisons of Sequential Interaction Patterns in Therapy of Experienced and Inexperienced Clinicians in the Parameters of Articulation, Delayed Language, Prosody, and Voice Disorders. Doctoral Dissertation, University of Denver, Denver, Colo. (1972).

Olsen, H.; Barbour, C.; and Michalak, D., *The Teaching Clinic.* Washington, D.C.: Publications-Sales Selection, National Education Association, 1201 Sixteenth Street, N.W. 20036 (1971).

O'Neill, J., and Peterson, H., The Use of Closed Circuit Television in a Clinical Speech Training Program. *Asha,* 6, 445-447 (1964).

O'Toole, T., Supervision of the Clinical Trainee. *Lang. Speech Hearing Serv. Schools,* 4, 132-139 (1973).

Paisley, T., Can Communication Research Help? Paper presented at the International Communication Association Convention, Montreal, Canada (1973).

Paisley, W., Identifying the Unknown Communicator in Painting and Music: The Significance of Minor Encoding Habits. *Journal of Communication,* 14, 219-237 (1964).

Pannbacker, M., Bibliography for Supervision. *Asha,* 17, 105 (1975a).

————————: Diagnostic Report Writing. *Journal of Speech and Hearing Disorders,* 40, 367-379 (1975b).

Parakh, J., A Study of Relationships Among Teacher Behavior, Pupil Behavior, and Pupil Characteristics in High School Biology Classes. (Project No. 7-1-22, Grant No. OEG 1-7-070022-3493). Bellingham, Wn.: Western Washington State College (1967).

Payne, P., and Gralinski, D., Effects of Supervisory Style and Empathy Upon Counselor Learning. *Journal of Counseling Psychology,* 15, 517-521 (1968).

Payne, P., and Koeller, D., Teaching and Supervising Student Clinicians Using Closed Circuit Television. Paper presented at the American Speech and Hearing Association Convention, Las Vegas, Nev. (1974).

Pearce, W., and Conklin, F., Nonverbal Vocalic Communication and Perception of a Speaker. *Speech Monographs,* 38, 235-241 (1971).

Perkins, W., Our Profession: What Is It? *Asha,* 4, 339-344 (1962).

Perkins, W., and Curlee, R., Causality in Speech Pathology. *Journal of Speech and Hearing Disorders,* 34, 231-238 (1969).

Perlis, L., The Volunteer. *Hearing and Speech Action,* 43, 24-27 (1975).

Pittenger, R.; Hockett, C.; and Danehy, J., *The First Five Minutes*. Ithaca, N.Y.: Martineau (1960).

Popham, W. (Ed.), *Criterion-Referenced Measurement: An Introduction*. Englewood Cliffs, N.J.: Educational Technology Publications (1971).

Poser, E., Training Behavior Therapists. *Behavior Research and Therapy*, 5, 37-41 (1967).

Powers, G., Asha Committee Report on Proposed Minimum Requirements for ETB Accreditation. *Asha*, 16, 627-629 (1974).

Powers, M., What Makes an Effective Public School Speech Therapist? *J. Speech Hearing Dis.*, 21, 461-467 (1956).

Prather, E., Standards for Quality Supervision of Clinical Practicum. In Miner, A. (Ed.), A Symposium: Improving Supervision of Clinical Practicum. *Asha*, 9, 471-481 (1967).

Prescott, T., The Development of a Methodology for Describing Speech Therapy. Doctoral Dissertation, University of Denver, Denver, Colo. (1970).

Prescott, T., and Tesauro, P., A Method for Describing Clinical Interaction With Aurally Handicapped Children. Paper presented at the American Speech and Hearing Association Convention, San Francisco, Calif. (1972).

——————————: A Method for Qualification and Description of Clinical Interactions with Aurally Handicapped Children. *J. Speech Hearing Dis.*, 39, 235-243 (1974).

Price, H., and Weston, A., Factors Perceived as Important in the Training of Clinicians: Producers vs. Consumers. Paper presented at the American Speech and Hearing Association Convention, Las Vegas, Nev. (1974).

Professional Services Board of the American Boards of Examiners in Speech Pathology and Audiology, *Accreditation of Professional Services Programs in Speech Pathology and Audiology*. Washington, D.C.: American Speech and Hearing Association (1974).

Pronovost, W.; Wells, C.; Gray, D.; and Sommers, R., Research: Current Status and Needs. *J. Speech Hearing Dis.*, Mono. Supp. 8, 114-123 (1961).

Ptacek, P., Supportive Personnel as an Extension of the Professional Worker's Nervous System. *Asha*, 9, 403-405 (1967).

Ptacek, P.; Black, J.; Hyman, M.; and Jenkins-Lee, J., A survey of the Functions, Uses, and Training of Specialized Personnel in Speech and Hearing. *Asha*, 15, 640-645 (1973).

Rabow, J., Quantitative Aspects of the Group-Psychotherapist; Role Behavior: A Methodological Note. *J. Soc. Psychol.*, 67, 31-37 (1965).

Raths, J., and Leeper, R., *The Supervisor: Agent for Change in Teaching*. Washington, D.C.: Association for Supervision and Curriculum Development, NEA, 1201 Sixteenth Street, N.W. (1966).

Rees, M., and Smith, G., Some Recommendations for Supervised School Experience for School Clinicians. *Asha*, 10, 93-104 (1968).

Reik, T., *Listening with the Third Ear*. New York: Farrar, Strauss and Giroux, Inc. (1948).

Rein, I., *Rudy's Red Wagon: Communication Strategies in Contemporary Society*. Glenview, Ill.: Scott, Foresman and Company (1972).

Reitz, J., Leadership and Group Effectiveness. In Anderson, J. (Ed.), *Supervision of Speech and Hearing Programs in the Schools*. Bloomington, Ind.: Indiana University (1970).

Richardson, S., Accountability to the Child with a Disorder of Communication. *Asha*, 16, 3-6 (1974).

Rippey, A. (Ed.), *Evaluating Student Teaching, a Forward Look at Theories and Practices*. Dubuque, Iowa: Wm. C. Brown Co., Inc. (1960).

Riskin, J., Family Interaction Scales: A Preliminary Report. *Archi. of Gen. Psych.*, 11, 484-494 (1964).

Roberts, W., Modes of Communication: A Model for Studying Teacher-Student Interaction. Doctoral Dissertation, Princeton Theological Seminary, Princeton, N.J. (1968).

Robertson, J., Supervision of Speech and Hearing Clinicians. Paper presented at the American Speech and Hearing Association Convention, Chicago, Ill. (1971).

Rogers, C., The Interpersonal Relationship: The Core of Guidance. *Harvard Educational Review*, 32, 416-429 (1962).

Rogers, C.; Gendlin, G.; Kiesler, D.; and Traux, C., *The Therapeutic Relationship and Its Impact: A Study of Psychotherapy with Schizophrenics*. Madison, Wisc.: University of Wisconsin Press (1967).

Rosenfeld, H., Instrumental Affiliative Functions of Facial and Gestural Expressions. *Journal of Personality and Social Psychology*, 4, 65-72 (1966).

Rosenhan, D., and Greenwald, J., The Effects of Age, Sex, and Socio-Economic Class on Responsiveness of Two Classes of Verbal Reinforcement. *Journal of Personality*, 33, 108-121 (1965).

Ross, M., Classroom Acoustics and Speech Intelligibility. In Katz, J. (Ed.), *Handbook of Clinical Audiology*. Baltimore, Md.: Williams and Wilkens (1972).

Ross, M., and Giolas, T., The Effect of Three Classroom Listening Conditions on Speech Intelligibility. *Am. Ann. Deaf*, 116, 580-584 (1971).

Roth, B., Clinical Accountability. A Symposium for the Systematic Analysis of Behavioral Interactions. In Turton, L. (Ed.), *Proceedings of a Workshop on Supervision in Speech Pathology. Institute for the Study of Mental Retardation and Related Disabilities*. Ann Arbor, Mich.: The University of Michigan, Continuing and Adult Education Unit, 29-40 (1973).

———————————: Research Needs in Supervision. In Turton, L. (Ed.), *Proceedings of a Workshop on Supervision in Speech Pathology*. Ann Arbor, Mich.: University of Michigan (1974).

Rousey, C., and Holzman, P., Recognition of One's Own Voice. *J. Personality Soc. Psychol.*, 6, 464-466 (1967).

———————————: Some Effects of Listening to One's Own Voice Systematically Distorted. *Percept. Motor Skills*, 27, 1303-1313 (1968).

Ruesch, J., and Kees, W., *Nonverbal Communication*. Berkeley and Los Angeles, Calif.: University of California Press (1956).

Ryan, B., The Use of Videotape Recording (VTR) in University Speech Pathology and Audiology Training Centers. *Asha*, 12, 555-556 (1970).

Sainesbury, P., A Model of Recording Spontaneous Movements by Time-Sampling Motion Pictures. *Journal of Mental Science*, 100, 742-748 (1954).

Salomon, G., and McDonald, F., Pretest and Posttest Reactions to Self-Viewing One's Teaching Performance on Video Tape. *Journal of Educational Psychology*, 61, 280-286 (1970).

Sanders, L., *Evaluation of Speech and Language Disorders in Children*. Danville, Ill.: Interstate Printers and Publishers (1972).

Sarno, M.; Silverman, M.; and Sands, Speech Therapy and Language Recovery in Severe Aphasia. *J. Speech Hearing Res.*, 13, 607-623 (1970).

Sathre, F.; Olson, R.; and Whitney, C., *Let's Talk*. Glenview, Ill.: Scott, Foresman, and Company (1973).

Schalk, M., Consistency and Reliability of Supervisory Evaluations at University Training Centers. Paper presented at the American Speech and Hearing Association Convention, San Francisco, Calif. (1972).

Scheflan, A., Natural History Method in Psychotherapy: Communicational Research. In *Methods of Research in Psychotherapy*. Edited by Gottschalk, L., and Auerback, A. New York: Appleton-Century-Crofts (1966).

Scheidel, T., *Speech Communication and Human Interaction*. Glenview, Ill.: Scott, Foresman and Company (1972).

Schmidt, J., Evaluating Student's Performance in Clinical Practicum. *North Dakota Speech and Hearing Journal*, 15, 40-59 (1972).

Schmidt, P.; Quigley, S.; and Quadagno, J., *Supervisors and Supervision of Teachers of the Deaf*. Champaign, Ill.: Institute for Research on Exceptional Children (1968).

Schubert, A.; Baird, J.; and Bowes, J.; A Study of Nonverbal Communication and Leadership in Task Oriented and Informal Small Groups. Paper distributed at the International Communication Association Convention, New Orleans, La. (1974).

Schubert, G., *The Analysis of Behavior of Clinicians (ABC) System (2nd Edition)*. Grand Forks, N.D.: University of North Dakota (1974a).

——————————: Suggested Minimal Requirements for Clinical Supervision. *Asha*, 16, 305 (1974b).

——————————: Hiring Certified Teachers as Teacher Aides: A Point of View. Paper presented at the Minnesota Speech and Hearing Association Convention, Alexandra, Minn. (1974c).

——————————: Evaluation of Clinical Practicum in Speech and Hearing Pathology. *North Dakota Speech Hearing J.*, 11, 1-12 (1968).

——————————: Higher Education and the Public School Speech Clinician. *Language, Speech and Hearing Services in Schools* (1975).

——————————: Supervision of Clinical Practice. *North Dakota Speech Hearing J.*, 10, 1-4 (1967).

Schubert, G., and Aitchison, C., A Profile of Clinical Supervisors in College and University Speech and Hearing Training Programs. *Asha*, 17, 440-447 (1975).

Schubert, G., and Glick, A., A Comparison of Two Methods of Recording and Analyzing Student Clinician-Client Interaction. *Acta Symbolica*, 5, 39-56 (1974).

Schubert, G., and Gudmundson, P., Effects of Videotape Feedback and Interaction Upon Nonverbal Behavior of Student Clinicians. Paper presented at the American Speech and Hearing Association Convention, Houston, Texas (1976).

Schubert, G., and Laird, B., The Length of Time Necessary to Obtain a Representative Sample of Clinician-Client Interaction. *The Journal of the National Student Speech and Hearing Association*, 3, 26-32 (1975).

Schubert, G., and Mercer, A., Nonverbal Behaviors Used by Two Different Groups of Clinicians During Therapy. *Acta Symbolica* 6, 41-57 (1975).

Schubert, G., and Miner, A., An Interaction Analysis System for Identifying the Behavior of Speech and Language Clinicians. Paper presented at the American Speech and Hearing Association Convention, New York, N.Y. (1970).
——————————: Modification of the Flanders' Interaction Analysis Categories for Observation in Speech Therapy. Paper presented at the American Speech and Hearing Association Convention, Chicago, Ill. (1971).
Schubert, G.; Miner, A.; and Prather, E., A Comparison of Student Clinicians' Behaviors as Measured by the Analysis of Behaviors of Clinicians (ABC) System. Paper presented at the American Speech and Hearing Association Convention, San Francisco, Calif. (1972).
Schubert, G.; Miner, A.; and Till, J., *The Analysis of Behavior of Clinicians (ABC) System.* Grand Forks, N.D.: University of North Dakota (1973).
Schubert, G., and Nelson, J., An Analysis of Verbal Behaviors Occurring in Speech Pathology Supervisory Sessions. *The Journal of the National Student Speech and Hearing Association,* 4, 17-26 (1976).
Schultz, M., The Bases of Speech Pathology and Audiology: What Are Appropriate Models? *Journal of Speech and Hearing Disorders,* 37, 118-122 (1972a).
——————————: *An Analysis of Clinical Behavior in Speech and Hearing.* Englewood Cliffs, N.J.: Prentice Hall (1972b).
Sevener, G., A Consistency Based Clinical Practicum Experience Using Systematic Planning with Evaluation Criteria for Accountability. Paper presented at the American Speech and Hearing Association Convention, Las Vegas, Nev. (1974).
Shannon, A., Facial Expression of Emotion: Recognition Patterns in Schizophrenics and Depressives. *Proceedings: 1971 ANA Research Conference.* New York: American Nurses' Association (1971).
Shelton, R., Therapeutic Exercise and Speech Pathology. *Asha,* 5, 855-859 (1963).
Shelton, R.; Arndt, W.; and Elbert, M., A Task for Evaluation of Articulation Change: I. Development of Methodology. *J. Speech Hearing Res.,* 10, 281-288 (1967a).
——————————: A Task for Evaluation of Articulation Change: II. Comparison of Task Scored During Baseline and Lesson Series Testing. *J. Speech Hearing Res.,* 10, 578-585 (1967b).
Shelton, R.; Hahn, E.; and Morris, H., Diagnosis and Therapy. In Spriestersbach, D., and Sherman, D. (Eds.), *Cleft Palate and Communication.* N.Y.: Academic Press (1968).
Sherman, D., Clinical and Experimental Use of the Iowa Scale of Severity of Stuttering. *Journal of Speech and Hearing Disorders,* 17, 316-320 (1952).
Sherman, D., and Moodie, C., Four Psychological Scaling Methods Applied to Articulation Defectiveness. *Journal of Speech and Hearing Disorders,* 20, 352-358 (1955).
Short, R., The Relationship of Teachers' Classroom Behavior to the Achievement of Junior High School Students and the Effect of Interaction Analysis Feedback on Teachers' Classroom Behavior. Doctoral Dissertation, University of Washington, Seattle, Wn. (1968).

Shriberg, L., Development of an Articulation Scoring Training Program (ASTP). Paper presented at the American Speech and Hearing Association Convention, San Francisco, Calif. (1972).
──────────: A Program for Evocation of /ɝ/. *J. Speech Hearing Dis.*, 40, 92-105 (1975).
Shriberg, L.; Filley, F.; Hayes, D.; Kwialkowski, J.; Schatz, J.; Simmons, K.; and Smith, M., The Wisconsin Procedure for Appraisal of Clinical Competence (W-PACC): Model and Date. *Asha*, 17, 158-165 (1975).
Simon, A., and Agazarian, Y., *Sequential Analysis of Verbal Interaction (SAVI)*. Philadelphia, Penn.: Research for Better Schools, Inc. (1967).
Simon, A., and Boyer, E., (Eds.), *Mirrors of Behavior*. Philadelphia, Penn.: Research for Better Schools, Inc. (1967).
Simon, C., To Summarize is to Focus: Consideration of a Method for Communicating Supervisory Comments to Student-Clinicians. Paper presented at the American Speech and Hearing Association Convention, Washington, D.C. (1975).
Simoni, F., A Proposed Model for Evaluating Clinical Performance. *J. of the Minnesota Speech and Hearing Association*, 12, 117-125 (1973).
Skinner, B., *Verbal Behavior*. New York: Appleton-Century-Crofts (1957).
Sloane, H., and MacAulay, B., *Operant Procedures in Remedial Speech and Language Training*. Boston, Mass.: Houghton Mifflin (1968).
Smith, K., and Larson, L., Minimum Clinical Competence for Speech Pathology School Practicum. Paper presented at the American Speech and Hearing Association Convention, Washington, D.C.: (1975).
Smith, R., and Flenning, F., Need for Approval and Susceptibility to Unintended Social Influence. *Journal of Consulting and Clinical Psychology*, 30, 383-385 (1971).
Smith, W., *Group Problem-Solving Through Discussion*. New York: Bobbs-Merrill Co., Inc. (1965).
Snyder, W., and June, B., *Psychotherapy Relationship*. New York: The Macmillan Co. (1961).
Solomon, D., and Yaeger, J., Effects of Content and Intonation on Perceptions of Verbal Reinforcers. *Perceptual and Motor Skills*, 28, 319-327 (1969a).
──────────: Determinants of Boy's Perceptions of Verbal Reinforcers. *Developmental Psychology*, 1, 637-645 (1969b).
Sommers, R.; Schaeffer, M.; Leiss, R.; Gerber, A.; Broug, M.; Fondrella, D.; Olson, J., and Tomkins, E., The Effectiveness of Group and Individual Therapy. *Journal of Speech and Hearing Research*, 9, 219-225 (1966).
Spear, P., Motivational Effects of Praise and Criticism on Children's Learning. *Developmental Psychology*, 3, 124-132 (1970).
Spear, P., and Spear S., Social Reinforcement Discrimination Learning and Retention in Children. *Developmental Psychology*, 7, 220 (1972).
Spriestersbach, D., As I See It--Clinician: A Status Title. *Asha*, 7, 464 (1965).
Stace, A., and Drexler, A., Special Training for Supervisors of Student Clinicians: What Private Speech and Hearing Centers Do and Think About Training Their Supervisors. *Asha*, 11, 318-320 (1969).
Starkweather, C., Behavior Modification in Training Speech Clinicians: Procedures and Implications. *Asha*, 16, 607-611 (1974).

Stech, E., Base Rate of Reinforcer Use in Clinical Practice: Inventory Modulation, and Frequency of Use of Reinforcers in Speech Pathology. Paper presented at the American Speech and Hearing Association Convention, Chicago, Ill. (1971).

Stech, E., Curtiss, J.; Troesch, P.; and Binnie, C., Clients' Reinforcement of Speech Clinicians: A Factor-Analytic Study. *Asha*, 15, 287-289 (1973).

Stevens, C., A Comparison of Nonverbal Behaviors of Beginning Clinicians and Advanced Clinicians. Master's thesis, University of North Dakota, Grand Forks, North Dakota (1976).

Stevens, N., The Moral Obligation to be Intelligible. *Scientific Monthly*, 70, 111-115 (1950).

Stinson, J., and Robertson, J., Follower-Maturity and Preference for Leader-Behavior Style. *Psychol. Rep.*, 32, 247-250 (1973).

Stoicheff, M., Motivating Instructions and Language Performance of Dysphasic Subjects. *Journal of Speech and Hearing Disorders*, 3, 75-85 (1960).

Stoller, F., Closed Circuit Television and Videotape for Group Psychotherapy with Chronic Mental Patients. *Amer. Psychol.*, 22, 158-162 (1967).

——————————: Focused Feedback With Videotape: Extending the Groups Function. In Gradza, G. (Ed.), *Innovations to Group Psychotherapy*. Springfield, Ill.: Charles C. Thomas (1968).

Strom, P., and Schubert, G., Comparison of Two Supervisory Conditions. *North Dakota Speech and Hearing Journal*, 16, 38-59 (1973).

Strong, B., Public School Speech Technicians in Minnesota. *Language, Speech and Hearing Services in the Schools*, 53-56 (1972).

Strunk, W., and White, E., *The Elements of Style*. New York: Macmillan (1959).

Taylor, M., A Measurement of Functional Communication in Aphasia. *Archs, Psys. Med. Rehabil.*, 88, 101-107 (1965).

Thompson, E. (Ed.), *Standard Nomenclature of Diseases and Operations. (5th Edition)* New York: McGraw-Hill (1961).

Till, J., The Use and Misuse of Evaluation Forms. *The Journal of the National Student Speech and Hearing Association*, 4, 48-53 (1976).

Trager, G., Paralanguage: A First Approximations. *Studies in Linguistics*, 13, 1-12 (1958).

Trelease, S., *How to Write Scientific and Technical Papers*. Cambridge, Mass.: MIT Press (1958).

Truax, C., Effective Ingredients in Psychotherapy: An Approach to Unraveling the Patient-Therapist Interaction. *Journal of Counseling Psychology*, 10, 256-263 (1963).

Truax, C., and Carkhuff, R., For Better or For Worse: The Process of Psychotherapeutic Personality Change. Paper read at Academic Assembly on Clinical Psychology, McGill University, Montreal, Canada (1963).

——————————: *Toward Effective Counseling and Psychotherapy: Training and Practice*. Chicago, Ill.: Aldine Publishing Company (1967).

Truax, C.; Carkhuff, R.; and Kodman, F., Jr., Relationships Between Therapist-Offered Conditions and Patient Change in Group Psychotherapy. *Journal of Clinical Psychology*, 21, 327-329 (1965).

Truax, C., and Mitchell, K., Research on Certain Therapist Interpersonal Skills in Relation to Process and Outcome. In Allen, Bergin, and Garfield, S., (Eds.), *Handbook of Psychotherapy and Behavior Change: An Empirical Analysis*. New York: John Wiley & Sons, Inc. (1971).

Truax, C., and Wargo, D., Antecedents to Outcome in Group Psychotherapy with Juvenile Client Self-Exploration. Unpublished Manuscript. Arkansas Rehabilitation Research and Training Center, University of Arkansas, Little Rock, Ark. (1967).

Turton, L. (Ed.), *Proceedings of a Workshop on Supervision in Speech Pathology.* Ann Arbor, Mich.: University of Michigan (1974).

Underwood, J., Interaction Analysis Between the Supervisor and the Speech and Hearing Clinician. Doctoral Dissertation, University of Denver, Denver, Colo. (1973).

——————————: *Underwood Category System for Analyzing Supervisor-Clinician Behavior.* University of Northern Colorado, Greeley, Colo. (1974).

United States Department of Health, Education, and Welfare, Office of Education, *The Utilization of Supportive Personnel in Speech Correction in the Public Schools: A Pilot Project.* Washington, D.C. (1970).

Utterback, W., *Group Thinking and Conference Leadership.* New York: Holt, Rinehart and Winston, Inc. (1964).

Van Hagen, C., *Report Writers Handbook.* Englewood Cliffs, N.J.: Prentice-Hall (1961).

Van Hattum, R., The Defensive Speech Clinicians in the Schools. *J. Speech Hearing Dis.,* 31, 234-240 (1966).

——————————: Services of the Speech Clinician in Schools: Progress and Prospect. *Asha,* 18, 59-63 (1976).

Van Riper, C., *Speech Correction: Principles and Methods,* 4th Ed. Englewood Cliffs, N.J.: Prentice-Hall (1963).

——————————: Success and Failure in Speech Therapy. *Journal of Speech and Hearing Disorders,* 31, 276-279 (1966).

——————————: Supervision of Clinical Practice. *Asha,* 7, 75-77, (1965).

Van Riper, C., and Dopheide, W., Diagnostic Services in a Training Center. *Asha,* 8, 37-39 (1966).

Ventry, I.; Newman, P.; and Johnson, K., The 1964 Membership of ASHA--Survey Results. *Asha,* 7, 219-230 (1965).

——————————: Personal Incomes in the Speech and Hearing Profession: Academic Faculty. *Asha,* 6, 67-73 (1964a).

——————————: Some Characteristics of ASHA Members Employed in College and University Speech and Training Programs. *Asha,* 6, 229-237 (1964b).

Verplanck, W., The Control of the Content of Conversation: Reinforcement of Statements of Opinions. *Journal of Abnormal and Social Psychology,* 51, 668-676 (1955).

Villarreal, J. (Seminar Ed.), *Seminar on Guidelines For Supervision of Clinical Practicum in Programs of Training for Speech Pathologists and Audiologists.* Washington, D.C.: American Speech and Hearing Association (1964).

Villarreal, J., and Lawrence, C., Undergraduate Preparation for Professional Education in Speech Pathology and Audiology: A Summary Report of a Conference. *Asha,* 11, 539-542 (1969).

Vine, I., Judgment of Direction of Gaze: An Interpretation of Discrepant Results. *British Journal of Social and Clinical Psychology,* 10, 320-331 (1971).

Wachtel, P., An Approach to the Study of Body Language in Psychotherapy. *Psychotherapy*, 4, 97-100 (1967).

Wagner, C., (Project Coordinator), *Conference on Standards for Supervised Experience for Speech and Hearing Specialists in Public Schools.* Orange County, Calif.: Orange County Board of Ed. (1969).

Walmon, M., Observing the Classroom Action System. *J. of Teacher Ed.*, 12, 466-470 (1961).

Walz, G., and Johnson, J., Counselors Look at Themselves on Videotape. *Journal of Counseling Psychology*, 10, 232-236 (1963).

Ward, L., and Webster, E., The Training of Clinical Personnel: I. Issues in Conceptualization. *Asha*, 7, 38-40 (1965a).

————————: The Training of Clinical Personnel: II. A Concept of Clinical Preparation. *Asha*, 7, 103-106 (1965b).

Watson, O., and Graves, T., Quantitative Research in Proxemic Behavior. *American Anthropologist*, 68, 971-985 (1966).

Weston, A., and Rousey, C., Voice Confrontation in Individuals with Normal and Defective Speech Patterns. *Percept. Motor Skills*, 30, 187-190 (1970a).

————————: The Use of a Tape Recorder in Clinical Practice. *Asha*, 12, 551-552 (1970b).

Willis, C., and Willis, J., Survey of Training Programs in Speech Pathology and Audiology. *Asha*, 16, 200-202 (1974).

Winitz, H., and Preisler, L., Effect of Distinctive Feature Pretraining in Phoneme Discrimination Learning. *J. of Speech and Hearing Res.*, 10, 515-530 (1967).

Wolfe, W., Preprofessional Education in Speech Pathology and Audiology VII. Oberlin College. *Asha*, 14, 170-171 (1969).

Wolfle, D., Bad Writing. *Science*, 155, 37 (1967).

Wood, K., Terminology and Nomenclature. In Travis, L. (Ed.), *Speech Pathology*. New York: Appleton-Century-Crofts (1957, 1971).

Woodford, F., Sounder Thinking Through Clearer Writing. *Science*, 156, 734-745 (1967).

Wright, E., *Interaction in the Mathematics Classroom: A Sub-Project Report of the Secondary Mathematics Evaluation Project.* (Technical Report No. 67-5). St. Paul, Minn.: Minn. National Laboratories, Minnesota State Dept. of Ed. (1967).

Yenawine, G., and Arbuckle, D., Study of the Use of Videotape and Audiotape as Techniques in Counselor Education. *Journal of Counseling Psychology*, 18, 1-6 (1971).

Zajonc, R., The Effects of Feedback and Probability of Group Success on Individual and Group Performance. *Human Relations*, 15, 149-161 (1962).

Zigler, E., and Kanzer, P., The Effectiveness of Two Classes of Verbal Reinforcers on the Performance of Middle- and Lower-Class Children. *Journal of Personality*, 30, 157-163 (1962).

# ADDITIONAL REFERENCES

Baldes, R.; Goings, R.; Herbold, D.; Jeffrey, R.; Wheeler, G.; and Frelinger, J., Supervision of Student Speech Clinicians. *Lang. Speech Hearing Serv. Schools*, 8, 76-84 (1977).

Chapey, R., and Chapey, G., Supervision: A Case Study. *Lang. Speech Hearing Serv. Schools*, 8, 256-263 (1977).

Gerstman, H., Supervisory Relationships: Experiences in Dynamic Communication. *Asha*, 19, 527-529 (1977).

Irwin, R., Microcounseling Interviewing Skills of Supervisors of Speech Clinicians. *Human Communication*, 4, 5-9 (1975).

Monnin, L., and Peters, K., Problem Solving Supervised Experience in the Schools. *Lang. Speech Hearing Serv. Schools*, 8, 99-106 (1977).

Mowrer, D., *Methods of Modifying Speech Behavior: Learning Theory in Speech Pathology*. Columbus, Ohio: Charles E. Merrill Publishing Co. (1977).

Pickering, M., An Examination of Concepts Operative in the Supervisory Process and Relationship. *Asha*, 19, 607-610 (1977).

Oratio, A., *Supervision in Speech Pathology: A Handbook for Supervisors and Clinicians*. New York: University Park Press (1977).

Oratio, A., A Factor-Analytic Study of Criteria for Evaluating Student Clinicians in Speech Pathology. *Journal of Communicative Disorders*, 9, 199-210 (1976).

Oratio, A., The Clinician's Level of Training as a Factor in Supervisors' Evaluations of Clinical Performance. *Ohio Journal of Speech and Hearing*, 12, 32-38 (1976).

Schubert, G., and Lyngby, A., The Clinical Fellowship Year (CFY). *The Journal of the National Student Speech and Hearing Association*, 5, 22-28 (1977).

Shriberg, L.; Filley, F.; Hayes, D.; Kwiatkowski, J.; Schatz, J.; Simmons, K.; and Smith, M., The Wisconsin Procedure for Appraisal of Clinical Competence (W-PACC): Model and Data. *Asha*, 17, 158-165 (1975).

# AUTHOR INDEX

## A

Agazarian, Y., 36, 39
Aitchison, C., 8, 95
Altman, H., 37
Amidon, E., 36
Anderson, A., 39
Argyris, C., 39
Aschner, M., 36

## B

Boone, D., 40, 44, 64, 65
Bordeen, J., 116
Boyer, E., 34

## C

Clements, R., 38
Chester, S., 111, 112
Colucci, S., 131
Culatta, R., 131

## D

Deever, R., 38
Demeke, H., 38
Dittman, A., 118

## E

Egolf, B., 111, 112
Engel, D., 135

## F

Flanders, N., 34, 35, 40, 42, 44, 45

## G

Gallagher, J., 36
Gardner, J., 71
Gallaway, F., 136
Glick, A., 65
Goeffrey, V., 76
Goldberg, S., 64
Gudmundson, P., 122

## H

Halfond, M., 5
Ham, R., 135
Herbert, E., 38, 73
Hill, W., 38
Hunter, E., 36

## I

Irwin, J., 128

## J

Jason, H., 39
Jourard, S., 114, 117
June, B., 39

## K

Klinkhammer, G., 135
Krout, M., 121

## L

Laird, B., 64
Llewellyn, L., 118
Longabaugh, R., 39